CRNA STUDENT STUDY PACK:

3 Books in 1!

Survive CRNA School

CRNA Mnemonics

MORE CRNA Mnemonics

Chris Mulder, CRNA, MSN

Table of Contents

Survive CRNA School

A GUIDE TO SUCCESS AS A NURSE ANESTHESIA STUDENT

CHRIS MULDER, CRNA, MSN

1

About the Author

Growing up, I never knew I wanted to be a nurse anesthetist. Hell, I'd never even heard of it and probably couldn't pronounce it if I had. Just like most of my friends, I wanted to be a baseball player. Don't worry...of course I had a back-up career. I could always become an astronaut if things didn't work out as planned. After graduating high school, reality came crashing down all around me. I spent two years drifting through life at my local community college searching for my purpose in this world. When I transferred to the nearest state university, I was forced to finally suck it up and make a decision. I've always liked to write, which is why I chose to obtain a degree in English. Unfortunately, someone forgot to tell me that I would eventually need to make a living. I'm sure there are some decent jobs an English graduate can get, but I couldn't find them. If you're not Stephen King or J.K. Rowling, it can be very difficult to make any real money in that field.

After spending a couple of years in a cubicle, selling things that people didn't want, I decided it was time to make a change. A friend suggested that I look into nurse anesthesia as a possible option, so I decided to check it out. This was the first I'd heard of it, and I thought she was pulling my leg. I spent several weeks researching the profession and the requirements to make it happen. Since my degree was in English, you can probably imagine the amount of pre-requisites I had to catch up on to get into nursing school. I was fortunate enough to get into an accelerated BA/BS to BSN program on my first application. After nursing school, I started working as an RN in a Medical ICU. This experience only fortified my passion to become a CRNA. I loved titrating medications, making independent decisions, and helping patients and families get through a difficult time. After 3 years, I finally managed to work my way into CRNA School. I had hoped to get accepted quicker, but I think I needed that time to be truly prepared for what I was about to get myself into.

CRNA School was the most difficult challenge I've ever had to endure. It tested me mentally and physically, and there were many times that I questioned whether I made the right decision. I'm glad I hung in there, because I really enjoy what I do now. I currently work at a level I trauma center taking care of all types of patients in almost all types of cases. On a few rare occasions, I get to take care of a healthy patient. But most of them are very sick with several comorbidities. When I look back, it seems like just yesterday that I first stepped foot into the hospital as a nurse anesthesia student. At the same time, it seems like ages ago. I'm thankful for every difficult day I've gone through ever since deciding to become a CRNA. It has made me the person I am today, and I wouldn't change a thing. On second thought, I guess I could have done without a select few of those lectures!

Introduction

Your story might be similar to mine, or maybe you always knew that becoming a CRNA is what you wanted. Anesthesia school is almost guaranteed to be more difficult than you expect. You'll begin to understand what I mean when you are waist deep in textbooks, trying to keep your eyes open to study after your 9th day in a row of clinicals. The goal of this book is not to teach you anesthesia. You will get much more than you bargained for in your respective CRNA School. I'm not going to attempt to squeeze hundreds of texts, studies, and experiences into one short book. Instead, I will try to teach you some tips and tricks that might help you along the way, including how to deal with some of the emotional issues that might arise, how to study smarter, and how to interact with others in your field. I want you to be able to not only survive, but also thrive, over the next 2-3 years. Hopefully by the end of this book, you'll feel more prepared and confident to face the many challenges that are up ahead.

I decided to write this because I wish someone had shown me the ropes when I was a student. The scariest part of anything is the unknown, and I think you might all classify anesthesia school in the realm of the unknown.

While this book won't be able to tell you exactly what to expect, it will hopefully alleviate some of the concerns you have and answer some burning questions for you. Take the advice if you think it will help, or simply ignore it if you think I'm full of it. I know I don't have all the answers, but this is some of what I've learned in school and beyond. Feel free to skip around through the book as you please. I tried to separate it into sections that you can access quickly if you're just looking for specific information. If there is something you have a question about or would like further clarification on, please email me at contact@kickassnursing.com. If I left something out that you would like my opinion on, I would be happy to help as much as I can. I'm open to critique and suggestions for improvement, or you can just contact me to let me know how much the book sucks if you want.

Chapter One

You're in! Now you can relax (well, if you have some Xanax)

You finally did it! After years of hard work and preparation, you've managed to beat out many of your peers to claim one of the few seats available in CRNA School. So pat yourself on the back, because just getting a foot in the door is a huge hurdle to jump. But after you breathe that sigh of relief, get ready to put in some hard work. The attrition rate for student nurse anesthetists can reach upwards of 10%, or more for some programs. Not only am I going to teach you the things I learned when I was in CRNA School, but also some of the things I wish I would have learned. These strategies are not meant as a replacement for hard work and persistence. But hopefully they will help make things a little easier as you go through the long, difficult journey that lies ahead.

If you've made it to this point in your life, you've likely spent at least a couple of years in the ICU or ER as a registered nurse. You are the cream of the crop in your unit and are well respected by all of your peers. Many of you may have been charge nurses, supervisors, or administrators. Your new reality as a student may be a difficult one to accept, and it will definitely take some time getting used to being the low person on the totem pole. The sooner you're able to accept it however, the sooner you'll be able to move on to succeeding in anesthesia school. You are now on equal footing with all of your classmates, most of you coming from similar situations. All the respect you've earned over your successful career vanishes instantly the first time you walk into that classroom. That's not to say that you won't regain that respect, but you will be starting from scratch.

Keeping that in mind, never forget where you came from. Just the fact that you're in CRNA School shows what you've accomplished so far in your career. Thousands of applications are submitted to nurse anesthesia programs throughout the country, while only a fraction of them are accepted. So even though you are on the low end of the totem pole, it is a pretty strong totem pole that plenty of people would love to be a part of. There will be days that go by that test your patience and make you wonder why the heck you ever decided to put yourself through this. At times, you will feel incredibly small and may even want to cry. Stay grounded, but remember that you are a great nurse no matter what happens. No professor, preceptor, or anesthesiologist can take that away from you.

The first day of class may be a little overwhelming. You will be meeting the only people who can comprehend exactly what you are going through over the next 2-3 years. Everyone will be nervous, but try to make a good impression. Don't be a recluse like I was. Instead, make as many friends as you can as fast as possible. They can mean the small difference between becoming a CRNA and going back to the ICU. This is also a time when you meet some of your teachers, get your syllabus, and gain a general understanding of what's to come. Listen closely to the requirements and expectations for each class. Some important information might be given that isn't on the syllabus, so be sure to bring something to write with.

You will also be given a list of books, some of which are required and some which are simply suggestions. I would recommend getting every book on the list, and then find some more. You can never get enough information, and there is plenty out there. Some books will have conflicting data and different opinions. It's good to have a wide variety of resources so you can get the best information available. Anesthesia is constantly changing, just like every other discipline in healthcare. Because of this, textbooks alone will not be able to keep up with these changes. Recent articles and studies can be a great resource for the latest information. You should always try to keep up with the latest trends in anesthesia. Not only will they advance your knowledge base, they also give you good conversation starters with your preceptors.

Although studies and articles are great for clinical development, almost everything you get graded on in class will come from materials presented in the syllabus. Time is a very valuable asset in CRNA School, so try to focus on the task at hand. It's great to keep up on the latest in anesthesia, but don't skip required reading to get it done. So, if you are getting tested on material from Basics of Anesthesia, then the article about flow-volume loops can probably wait. If you have an exam tomorrow on antibiotics in Pharmacology, don't start reading the latest studies on ischemic optic neuropathy in the prone position. Flow-volume loops and blindness during a spinal fusion are great topics to learn about, but the information can be absorbed another day.

Chapter Two

Getting your textbooks

I'm sure I don't need to tell you how expensive textbooks can be. You probably have plenty of experience with this in your pursuit of a nursing degree. If you can afford it, just go ahead and get the books from the school bookstore. This will save you a lot of time and trouble in the long run, as it will ensure that you get the right book by the right author in the right edition. But as an SRNA without an income, you'll probably find it very important to make every penny count. No one would blame you if you decided to go another route. There are a few different options if you have to cut down on expenses in this area.

The first is to find them used on various web sites, such as eBay or Amazon. This has become very popular over the past few years, so there are several places to choose from. Some sites even act as a sort of liaison. For instance, at www.bigwords.com, you put the book information in the toolbar and it shows you all of the prices from various competitors. Shop around until you find the best deals. Just be careful, as some prices might be too good to be true. A really cheap textbook may have flaws, such as missing or ripped pages, lots of markings, etc. A book with a lot of writing and underlining in it may not seem like a big deal, but something like that can be very distracting when you are trying to focus on a specific topic.

You might also be able to buy some books very cheaply from upperclassmen or graduates of the program. Most students are running on empty towards the end of the program and right after graduation. They are looking for just about any way to make some extra money until they get that first paycheck. But again, if you go down this road, make sure the books are in the correct edition. Some of the textbooks are used again every semester, but they are often updated or changed entirely.

You could also rent your textbooks from sites like Chegg or Amazon. Make sure you search for your books by the ISBN number so you can make sure you have the correct one. I accidentally rented the British version of a textbook once in nursing school, and it made for a very difficult semester. Also, keep in mind that textbooks are usually rented by the semester. After the semester is over, you are required to send them back. I had to do this many times as I was running low on cash throughout the program. Later in the year, there was nothing I could do if I wanted to look back at something in the book. It would have been much more helpful for me to have all of my books when it came time to study for my comprehensive exams and boards.

The last option and one I would highly recommend against is that of sharing with your fellow classmates. It might seem like a good idea at first, but it will be a huge inconvenience as your program moves along. Unless you have the same schedules and always want to look at the same things, sharing will not be an easy task. You would have to sit next to each other in class with the book between the two of you, and you wouldn't be able to study exactly what you want whenever you wanted to. Anesthesia school is tough enough without having to worry about these types of silly things. It's just not worth the hassle to be able to save a little money. In short, whether they are new or used, buy your textbooks if you can. It will save you a huge headache in the long run.

Chapter Three

Finding a way to pay for it

Paying for school is probably something you've already gotten a handle on if you've come this far. However, I think it's a subject that deserves some attention. I wasn't sure how I was going to finance everything until just before school started. I just focused mainly on getting into school, and I decided to worry about the money later. Financing can become a huge issue in CRNA School because there are very few, if any, programs that allow you to work while in school. So not only do you need to find a way to pay for tuition and books, but you also have to think about basic living expenses and lost wages for 2-3 years.

The most obvious way to pay for all of this is through student loans. Graduate students are eligible for up to $20,500 per year in unsubsidized Direct Loans. Any additional amount, up to the cost of attendance, can be achieved by taking out government PLUS loans for a slightly higher interest rate. Cost of attendance includes tuition, books, and living expenses. However, the financial aid office of the specific school you are attending determines the cost of attendance, not the government. So this amount may vary for each student from school to school. Even with all of this assistance, sometimes it's still not enough. This is especially true if you are a single parent or someone with a spouse who stays at home.

There is also the option of private student loans, which are much harder to come by these days. They are difficult to find, but some are available if you have decent credit. You might run across the same problem as government loans in that they will often cover only up to the cost of attendance. I had to rely on these a lot more than I wanted to, and I am paying for it now. Do what you have to do if it comes down to it, but try to stay away from these higher interest loans.

Another way to get some financial assistance is by applying for those elusive scholarships. These are extremely difficult to find and you typically have to be an academic star to get these. But there are some that just about anyone can get. You might have to write something on a specific subject, put in a certain amount of volunteer hours, or complete some sort of research. Your school's financial aid office should be able to help you find some of these opportunities. You may also be able to find some at the AANA (American Association of Nurse Anesthetists) web site or your state's Anesthesia Association. But don't stop there. There are several scholarships available for any master's level degree, not just nurse anesthesia. Type in "master's scholarships" into any search engine and you'll see what I mean. With great persistence, I suppose it would be possible to find enough scholarship money to cover much of your tuition.

If you don't mind putting in some time for your country after graduation, you can get great financial help from the Army or Navy. In exchange for work after graduation, they will pay a monthly stipend to help cover your living expenses. The Army STRAP program now pays close to $2000 per month. They also offer student loan repayment to go along with this (up to $50,000 for reserves and $120,000 for active duty). It's a truly great thing to be able to give service to your country, but not everyone is cut out for it. Make sure this is something you are willing to commit to, as there is no going back once you sign. They will accept service in the form of active duty or reserves as a nurse anesthetist.

If the military isn't your thing, you could always look for anesthesia groups to pay for your tuition or give you a stipend each month. These are not easy to find, but there are still some out there. They will obviously want a commitment of some sort, so make sure you know what you are signing. You can call or email different groups to see if they would be interested in such an arrangement. The only catch is that they are usually looking for someone who has at least a year of anesthesia school under their belt. They also want someone who has decent grades and good clinical evaluations. Start your search at your own clinical sites. They already know your clinical skill and work ethic, and will be much more likely to work with you. Plus, it will be an easy transition when you graduate, going from an SRNA to a CRNA in the same place. Some people prefer to go somewhere different than their school's clinical site, fearing that they would be forever branded a "student" in the eyes of the anesthesiologists and other co-workers. When I graduated, I decided to stay at the same site, and I didn't find this to be an issue.

Chapter Four

Study smarter, not harder

You know the old saying, "you can't pick your parents?" Well the same holds true for your teachers. You are going to have some teachers that you love, while there will be others who you could easily do without. Unfortunately, these aren't undergraduate courses that you can simply withdraw from. Ah, how I longed for those days in undergrad when we had a drop/add week in the beginning of the semester. If you didn't like a class for any reason, you could simply drop it and add a different one. Well this isn't undergrad, so you're pretty much out of luck if you're not happy. Instead of lamenting this fact, try to make the most of every class and every teaching style.

Talk to your upperclassmen so you know what's coming. You don't want any surprises. You may be able to listen to certain teachers and everything will click as the words flow from their mouths. There will likely be others whose lectures you have to record and listen to over and over. Learn their teaching styles, but more importantly, learn their testing styles. Find out if they go strictly from their lectures and power points, or if random items from the textbook also show up on exams. Previous students should be able to help you some with this information, but it may take a test or two to figure out what they're looking for.

In the beginning, try to cover all your bases. For instance, if there is a reading assignment on the schedule, make sure you read it. Don't just look at the notes from the lecture and the PowerPoint. It is a lot of work at first, but you will find it easier to manage your time as each class progresses. Most professors will give you some idea of their expectations at the start of each semester. But you'll find that most will show certain tendencies on their exams. While you should always study everything that's on the syllabus, you will want to focus more of your energy covering these tendencies.

It is vitally important for you to find a way to study that works for you. It's going to be impossible to learn everything that is thrown at you in CRNA School. Are you an audio, visual, or kinesthetic type of learner? Unless you have a photographic memory, it would be helpful to determine whether you learn best by listening to a lecture, looking at pictures and video, or by physically doing something. Many people already know what kind of learner they are, but there are lots of tests out there to find out if you're not sure. As classes move along, you will be able to hone in on the things that help you recall all of the information given to you.

When I was in school, almost all of the lectures were video recorded along with the PowerPoint presentation the professors worked from. So we could essentially go back and re-take the lecture as often as we would like. Whether your school does this or not, I would highly recommend recording the audio from the lectures yourself. This way, you will always have the file to reference back to at any time. Many of my classmates would listen to these lectures whenever they were driving to and from class or clinicals. I tried this at first, but it never worked for me like it did for others. I would just find myself spacing out, thinking of much more interesting things while I drove. I ended up using that time to decompress a little, just listening to music or sports, trying not to think too much. Clearly, I needed more than just audio recordings to get me through.

In my school, every lecture was presented by way of PowerPoint. I personally found it very difficult to study directly from these PowerPoints. Instead, I converted them all to a Microsoft Word document, allowing the words to flow more like a story instead of window after window. I am not very tech savvy, so I had to go through slide after slide, copying a pasting each paragraph. Then I would manually re-format every sentence and picture. There must be an easier way to get this done, as it was very time consuming. If I had a few extra hours, I would sometimes transcribe the audio lecture into a word document also. This was usually a strategy reserved for those teachers that tested a lot of content from the lecture itself, information often left out of the PowerPoint or textbook itself. This was helpful during my first couple semesters, but became too difficult as I progressed in the program.

Something else that might work for you is to make questions and answers for the material. I used to go through every sentence of the PowerPoints, formulating a question and answer for each. They can be simple true/false questions, multiple choice, or direct answer. Just this process alone accounted for most of my absorption of the material. The work isn't just mindless formatting. You have to think of a way to arrange a question that would be fitting for the answer. Working through each question this way was one of the best studying techniques I utilized during the program. After I completed this, I would then take the questions and make flashcards out of them. You can make physical flashcards or create them online. There are also several apps that offer this function. Keep looking repetitively at 5-10 flash cards at a time, until you have them memorized, then move to the next. The idea is to work your way up to memorizing the entire stack.

These are great strategies, but many of them take up a lot of very valuable time, something which comes at a premium the further you move along in your program. Dividing the work will help immensely in saving you that precious time and energy. A good tip is to form a small group and have each person take turns transcribing audio, converting to Word, or making flashcards. You can set up a group web site for the entire class if you'd like, so everyone can post the things they've worked on. A couple of great sites for this are Quizlet and Dropbox. You could also get someone else to do some of the work for you. If you have the money, there are plenty of web sites that have freelancers who would love to transcribe audio or convert PowerPoints for a fee.

Mnemonics were also a huge help for me as I went through anesthesia school. There are several that are fairly well known, but you can make up just about anything that will help you remember. They don't even have to make sense, as long as they help you recall information better. For example, you might know one of the common mnemonics used to help you remember a basic set-up before any case. SOAPME was very useful during my first few months to help remember what I needed before starting any case. It stands for Suction, Oxygen, Airways (ET tube, LMA, etc), Positioning (proper padding, pillows, etc), Monitors/Meds, and Equipment. This is just one example of the hundreds I used while in school. Search for some on the internet or make some up on your own. It may seem silly, but they are a savior for many.

When it comes to studying, learn by trial and error. Repeat the techniques you used that helped you pass an exam, but discard the techniques that were a waste of time. You want to study smarter, not harder. You may not benefit from making flashcards or listening to recordings, but it would be a good idea to a least give it a try. When I was in school, I found myself grasping at anything that might give me some sort of advantage. If you find that you are acing your tests, then stick with whatever works. But if you think you could use a little help, try out some of the methods I mentioned.

Chapter Five

The classmate Advantage

When I was in school, I played sort of the loner role. At least I believe that's how my classmates saw me. I am married with 3 kids, and I value my time with them very much. Between classes and clinicals, I barely saw them as it was. Because of this, I ended up arriving to class right before it started, and I would leave as soon as it was over. Most of my classmates would hang around the classroom to chat or meet up somewhere to study. While they were quizzing each other for the pharmacology exam, I was quizzing my son for his geometry exam. I always studied alone, usually after everyone else in my house had already gone to sleep.

Although I wouldn't change the way I approached it, I know that it caused me to skate a lot closer to the edge than many of my peers. I would strongly suggest that you make friends with as many of your classmates as possible. Form study groups and bounce ideas off each other. When you might be confused with a subject, they might say just the right thing to help it all sink in. Also, I believe that all of the study methods mentioned before will likely stick in your mind the more your talk about them with other people. Besides that, studying alone is not a whole lot of fun. You can find yourself spinning, reading passages over and over, realizing each time you have no idea what you just read. Having someone else there to snap you out of it makes a huge difference when it comes time for the test.

In your class, there are going to be a few students at the top and a few at the bottom. But most of you will find yourselves somewhere in between. If you don't understand something, ask your classmate. They will either know the answer already, or they are having the same trouble and you can figure it out together. Just make sure you're always there when another classmate needs help from you. This symbiotic relationship also works well in clinicals. Talk to each other about your experiences. Share your successes, share your failures, and then share your failures again. It's great to hear how fantastic one of your classmates did in their first intubation attempt, and that information may help you a little. They can tell you about their technique and walk you through the steps. But it's even more valuable information to hear about the intubation they missed. Find out what happened, why it happened, and what they could have done differently.

You can't succeed in anything until you fail a little. Try to learn from other people's errors as much as you can. But don't think that you will avoid all mistakes. You are going to make a few (ok, you are going to make a lot of) mistakes. But that's all part of becoming a great CRNA. As long as you learn from your past and avoid those same mistakes in the future, then you won't have any problems. The CRNA's and anesthesiologists you work with were in your shoes at one time. They understand that you are there to learn, and most are very forgiving. When you slip up, acknowledge it, talk about it with your preceptor, and grow from it. You will gain much more from a bad day than you ever will from a good day. Don't forget to broadcast your mistakes to the rest of your classmates. They will appreciate it, just like you will when they tell you their stories.

Another great way to connect with your peers is by attending workshops and meetings offered by the AANA or your state's organization. These are excellent opportunities to meet other students and CRNAs from around the country. Often, you school will pay for you to attend or reimburse you. I wish I had attended more of these when I was a student. They give you the chance to see what things are like in anesthesia in places outside of your clinical site. We often get used to things in our little bubbles, but if you dare to venture out you will find that there are many more ways of doing things. Also, you can get an amazing amount of training with the latest products in anesthesia. There are workshops available for difficult airway, regional anesthesia, and learning the business side of anesthesia.

These are just a few options out there. During your time as an SRNA, try to keep track of when these things are offered and check with your school to see if it is something they'd be willing to foot the bill for.

Chapter Six

Setting up before cases

At the beginning of each day, I always start with my machine check. The newer machines require little more than pressing a few buttons, but you really should learn how to do a traditional check on an older machine. Once the machine is checked, make sure you have working suction. Many would suggest that this is the first thing you should always do, and maybe it is. The reason I do the machine check first is to get the process started. Since the newer machines have self-checks that take a few minutes, I do everything else while it's cooking. As long as the suction gets checked before you start a case, I'm not sure it matters when you do it. Next, I make sure there is adequate oxygen supply in the tank, just in case the wall supply malfunctions. I've never had to use it, but you never know. Then I make sure I have a working ambu bag and mask. Get your tape ready for the eyes and have the tape ready to secure the ET Tube once it's in place. The order you do these things doesn't matter as much as making sure they all get done. It's important to have a routine in place, doing the same steps in the same order every time. If you do this, it's much less likely that you'll forget something.

Once everything is checked, I always make an emergency set-up in addition to each specific case. I get a couple of different sized ET Tubes prepared, along with a variety of oral airways. I keep them covered and usually don't have to use them. But I always have them ready. Aside from emergencies, they may also come in handy if your tube accidentally gets dropped during intubation (as you can imagine, it's not really a good idea to pick up a tube from the ground and stick it into someone's trachea). Unfortunately, this has actually happened on occasion (not to me, of course!). But it wasn't a big deal because the backup tubes were already waiting in the wings. Trust me...the day you don't have them ready is the day you'll wish you had. I'm sure some of you remember being in the ICU with a patient you just didn't feel right about. You would bring the code cart in front of the room to ward off evil spirits. Well, it's the same idea for your emergency set-up.

After I have my back up supplies prepared and everything checked, I start setting up for the specific case I expect to be managing. For a general anesthesia case requiring intubation, I first make sure to put out the ET Tube. In my facility, we typically use a 7.0 ET Tube for a female and a 7.5 ET Tube for a male. If the patient is expected to stay intubated after the case, we will usually use an 8.0. The preference of the ET Tube size varies from site to site, so make sure you know the typical sizes used in your facility.

When setting up an ET Tube, first push the plastic connector into the tube itself to make sure it is snug. Put the stylet into the tube and bend it to preference. I personally prefer a hockey stick appearance with a small curve at the end. Make sure the stylet is not past the murphy's eye at the end of the tube. You can bend the top of the stylet near the connector to make sure it can't slip further down. Next, take a 10 cc syringe and test the pilot balloon to make sure there are no leaks. After this meets your satisfaction, withdraw all of the air back into the syringe.

Next to the ET tube, have your intubating blade of preference. I like to keep both of them out and next to each other. This way, if I am unsuccessful with one type of blade, I could make a second attempt with the other. Your anesthesiologist might prefer a different blade than you do also. You never know if they will have to intubate after your attempts. Near the tube and the blades, have an oral airway, a tongue depressor, and a soft bite block (made from rolled 4x4 gauze). Have something ready to monitor the patient's temperature. The esophageal probe is preferred, but you can also monitor with a nasopharyngeal probe, or skin probe. You might get lucky if the patient has a

Foley catheter in with a temperature probe attached. Also, have a couple of ekg pads to monitor twitches during paralysis.

For a general anesthesia case that calls for an LMA, the setup is a little different. Remember, no matter what type of anesthesia you're doing, you should always be prepared to intubate. Fortunately, this preparation was already done with your back up/emergency pack. Typical LMA sizes are 3 for a female, 4 for a male (or larger female), and 5 for a large male. You will see the typical suggested weight for each LMA size on the packaging. This is just a guide, and usually you can't determine an accurate size until you look at the patient. Lightly lubricate the outside of the cuff (not the part that will be facing the airway) and take out a few cc's of air. The amount of air you should take out is purely subjective. Some people take out all of the air, while others don't take any out. I think most CRNAs are somewhere in the middle, taking out just a little. Next to your LMA, have your oral airway, soft bite block, and tongue depressor. Just remember that an LMA will not protect against aspiration! You will be reminded of this approximately 500,000 times throughout your time as an SRNA, so don't forget it!

For a MAC (Monitored Anesthesia Care) case, you need to make sure you have a nasal cannula that will also monitor etCO2. These types of cases require a great deal of vigilance, as you have no airway protection. The patient is breathing on their own without an airway device, and your goal is to keep it this way. Have oral airways close by and have your suction even closer. As always, make sure you have an ET Tube and blade at the ready in case things go bad. It is never *just* a MAC, though you will hear this said many times. It generally takes a lot more skill to manage these types of cases than one in which an advanced airway is already in place.

Certain medications are drawn up for each specific case, but there are some standard things you will always want to have ready. First of all, succinylcholine is your friend. Keep it ready just in case. It can get you out of a jam in a hurry. You will also want to have some vasopressors ready in case of hypotension. Phenylephrine and Ephedrine are good choices, and the first ones most facilities use. Gylcopyrrolate is another great drug that should be ready to go in case of bradycardia. In my facility, these drugs are usually prepared ahead of time by the pharmacy. However, you will have to mix your own in some places. For starters, know how to mix Ephedrine and Phenylephrine. If Ephedrine is in the usual 50 mg/mL vial, then you would take 1 mL and add it to 9 mL of saline to result in a push concentration of 5 mg/mL. Phenylephrine is usually in a 10 mg/mL vial. Take 0.1 mL (1 mg) and add it to 9.9 mL of saline to reach a push concentration of 100 mcg/mL. Keep in mind that different facilities might use different concentrations. Of course, as always, make sure the typical emergency drugs, such as epinephrine and Atropine, are ready and available should the need present itself.

There are 2 blades most commonly used for intubation. These would be the curved Macintosh (Mac) and the straight Miller blade. A Mac is used to slide to the back of the tongue into the vallecula, which will lift the epiglottis indirectly to hopefully reveal a beautiful grade I view of the vocal cords. Conversely, the Miller blade is inserted under the epiglottis, lifting it directly to get the view you're looking for. It's really a matter of preference as to which blade you should use. It is typically a good idea to start out with the Mac as a student. It is more helpful in identifying anatomy and usually comes easier to most. Once you have done several intubations, you can start using the Miller more and more often. Most people will develop a favorite blade, but try to become proficient with both. While I can use the Miller if I need to, I feel more comfortable using the Mac blade. However, you will notice that many experienced clinicians will use the Miller almost exclusively.

Chapter Seven

Big Pimpin' (working with preceptors)

Preceptors will often quiz you during your time in clinicals with them. Sometimes the questions will be related to the case, while other times the questions are pulled from left field. This quizzing is commonly known in many SRNA circles as getting "pimped." Some of your preceptors are asking you these questions because they genuinely want to help advance your learning. Other preceptors are honestly just trying to figure out how far along your knowledge base is. Finally, there are some preceptors who simply get a kick out of watching you squirm. I think some of it has become the culture to give students a hard time. Many CRNAs weren't treated with kid gloves when they were in school either, and they view it as a rite of passage. I think a little tough love is necessary sometimes if it helps you grow as an anesthesia provider. But I don't think being mean for the sake of being mean is the right way to go about it.

I know it's going to be difficult, but please try not to think of getting pimped in a negative way. Believe it or not, the questions I remember most vividly from school didn't come from any lecture or exam. They came during intubations, line placements, and titrating of anesthesia. It can sometimes be very hard to stumble through question after question when you are struggling to just get the tube through the cords. But those questions and discussions during cases are the ones that will likely be forever burned in your memory. With that said, it would look much better for you to get a majority of these questions correct.

Make sure you know your stuff, especially the basics. You absolutely have to have your top-drawer meds memorized. This means dosing, onset, duration, method of action, and indications. If you've known in advance which case you are doing, you should know all of the anesthetic implications. You should know what to expect in the case, how much blood is lost on average, and things that you might need to do differently in comparison with other cases. Try to look up your patient's information well in advance of the case. This way, you can research their specific disease processes and know how it will impact the care you give them. You can look up their medications and determine if any of them affect your anesthetic plan also. It will be seen as inexcusable in many preceptors' eyes to miss those sorts of things if you've had time in advance to look everything up. Of course, there will be many times when you get a new case that you haven't had time to research. Your preceptor will be more understanding in this scenario, but you will need to learn to adapt to change and know how to find information on the fly.

If you don't know the answer to a question, try to start with something you do know that's related and work your way through it in your head. If you absolutely don't know something, then say so. But let your preceptor know that you will get back to them with an answer. Make sure you follow up on this! That night, research the topic and write about your findings. They are not expecting a novel here, but it should be more than a couple sentences. Make it look like you cared about what they were asking you. A couple paragraphs should suffice for most things. Try to find that preceptor the next morning to hand it to them or put it in their box. If they have time, see if they will discuss it with you. I would strongly suggest that you keep a file of questions you have been asked along with the answers. Our class kept a file titled "pimp questions" that could be accessed by all of the students. So if I knew I was going to be with a specific preceptor, I could look in that file to see what types of questions had been asked before by them.

On days you are with a preceptor, try to make a good impression. It goes beyond a flawless intubation and seamless wake up. No matter how well you do technically, it won't mean anything if you are difficult to work with. It's ok to be a little quiet. Sometimes that is preferred over some of the alternatives. However, try to be personable. When they aren't asking you questions, try to think of something good to ask them, or follow up on something they've already talked about. It will make you seem interested and involved in the case, which is much better than being disengaged. Make sure the questions you ask don't have obvious answers that you should already know. You may end up shooting yourself in the foot.

I would recommend that you don't ask the same question twice, even if it's directed to a different preceptor. It shows a definite lack of interest. Either you didn't care enough to remember what the answer was, or you were only asking because you wanted to *seem* interested. It may not be that big of a deal to most, but why take the chance? While we're on the subject, try to ask questions that will help you get better. Ask things like "do you have any pointers or tips to improve my intubation technique?" You might also ask something like "what are some of the different ways this could be done?" The point here is to make sure your preceptor knows that you aren't just there simply because you're on the schedule. Show them that you are interested and want to learn, and most will be more than happy to teach you.

It would also be a very good idea to have a general preceptor preferences file. You will quickly find out that every CRNA and anesthesiologist has a different way of doing things. Keep a detailed file on your computer of every preceptor you've been with. Remembering little things that each person does differently will go a long way. Although you might be with a new preceptor every day, they might only have a student once or twice a week. They are likely to remember the things they told you and the things you've discussed together. Keep track of things like where certain people like to keep their eye tape before induction: on the mask, on the machine, or somewhere else. Do they like to use a specific gas more than most? What is their preferred method to get patients breathing? Do they like to use a lot of narcotics? You get the idea.

In the end, it shouldn't matter how you do things, as long as there is a valid reason and it works. But it definitely will matter to most of your preceptors until you are much further along and they have gained a certain level of comfort working with you. I have a specific routine that keeps my mind right, as will most other CRNAs you are with. Everything is in the same spot for every case. If I have to reach for something quickly, I know exactly where it is because it's always there. Although every case is unique, there is a basic way I do my inductions, maintenance, and emergence. It's easy to get rattled if something is out of place or different in some way. So try not to get annoyed when your preceptor keeps redirecting you to do things their way. As you move further along as an SRNA, you are going to learn to take the good things you see and hopefully leave the bad. You will eventually have your own way of doing things. But when you are first getting started, try to learn what they want and duplicate it the next time you are with them. Encourage your classmates to do the same so you can share information with each other.

Chapter Eight

Maintaining confidence while getting the most out of your clinical time

Try to remember back to your first clinical day in nursing school. Most of you probably can still feel that very real urge to throw up. Well, your first day of clinicals in CRNA School will likely be much worse. At least it was for me. It took most of my first year before the butterflies in my stomach began to fade. This might not be a huge problem for some of you. But then again, I would frankly be concerned if you weren't the slight bit nervous. It shows that you're human and that you understand the seriousness of what you're getting yourself into. These patients are real and we hold their lives in our hands. Any mistakes or missteps can have disastrous consequences. This is something that you always need to remember no matter how far along you are in your career.

With that in mind, try to temper your nerves as much as possible. Even if you are scared as hell on the inside, show nothing but confidence on the outside. This will help tremendously to put your preceptors at ease, not to mention the patients and their families. It may sound strange, but the more they believe in you, the more you will believe in yourself. If your preceptors see the fear in your eyes, they will be more likely to look for flaws. They will probably ask you more questions to find out how much you really know. If you look like you know what you're doing, more often than not, they are happy to just let you do your thing.

Once you get over those initial butterflies and you've cleaned yourself up, try to stop running the other way when something unfamiliar presents itself. Use your time as a student CRNA wisely, and try to get as many experiences as possible. Don't be afraid of looking stupid, because now is the time to learn. It will look a lot worse if you don't know how to do something after you graduate. Ask your preceptors and attending doctors if you can get as many opportunities as possible. Watch central line placements enough times and then ask if you can try doing some. If your patient is a difficult intubation, ask if you can get a look with the fiber optic scope. Ask to get your hands on things even when your patient isn't a difficult intubation. Healthy patients with easy airways are good ones to learn things like the lightwand, bougie, Glidescope, fiberoptic, etc. Practice now so you will know how to use these things when they are really needed. Ask your preceptor if you can try using different medications or anesthetic techniques that you don't have much experience with. If there is an interesting case, see if you can go help out or at least observe. You are only an

SRNA once, so make the most of your time in school.

Don't worry about things like missing an intubation, having difficulty masking, difficulty putting in an a-line, etc. These are the things you will get better with every time you do it. While we're on the subject, I should clarify what I mean by "missed intubation." It can be defined in a few different ways. For example, you might struggle to get a good view, so you hand over the blade to your preceptor. If they are able to get a good view easily without doing much differently, I would consider that a miss. If you put the tube in the esophagus instead of the trachea, that's a clear miss. We would refer to that as "tubing the goose." Don't get discouraged by these times. They happen to everyone, even experienced CRNAs from time to time. During intubation, make sure you tell your preceptor or attending exactly what you see as you go. If you don't have a great view, let them know. Don't intubate blindly unless you are instructed to. If your preceptor thinks you have a good view, it is not going to go well if you tube the goose. On the other hand, if your preceptor allows you to try to intubate with a difficult view, then it won't look nearly as bad.

You are also going to have difficulty masking certain patients. I haven't met anyone that was an expert at masking their first day, or even their first couple of years. It's one of the hardest things in anesthesia to get down. Have your oral airway ready, but try to master it as much as you can without one. Watch other people mask and try to learn from them. Be sure to put your fingers on the jawbone, not the soft tissue. Lift the jaw towards the mask, rather than pressing down on the face. Lift the mask as needed to let some trapped air out, creating your own sort of pop-off valve. You're likely going to hear these same tips hundreds of times, but only because they will help you accomplish the lofty goal of achieving gas exchange in the lungs. Lastly, the only tried and true way to become very good at intubation and masking is by practice, over and over again. Failure isn't true failure when you're in anesthesia school. Sure, it hurts in the moment. But it's what makes you better in those same situations in the future.

Chapter Nine

Coming to terms with your new hectic schedule

.

I've heard many stories about CRNA students whose personal lives unravel a little while in school. It's hard to keep a relationship with your new busy schedule. Many end up breaking it off with girlfriends and boyfriends or getting divorced from their spouse. It's a sacrifice for your family as much as it is for you, if not even more so. When I started my anesthesia training, I was married with 2 small children. I'm happy to say that we stayed married through everything and even added a 3rd baby to the mix. But it was definitely a trying experience for all of us. My children had a hard time understanding why I had to stay late at the hospital, then come home and study all night. My wife knew what I was up against, but it still wasn't easy for her to accept some of our time apart.

Before you start school, have a long talk with your family. If you have children, be sure to include them in the discussion. Explain the specifics of what is required to get through the program. Make sure they understand that all of the time spent apart now is to prepare for a better future for all of you. On days before an exam, don't just go in your room or office and start studying. Spend a little time first telling them what you are doing and why. It will help, but it certainly won't fill that void you've left.

Lots of hard work and dedication are required to finish CRNA School, but you can't forget about the very people you're doing it for. Take a night off from studying here and there. Spend a weekend at the beach every once in a while. Make a date at the movies with your significant other. Hard work is necessary, but enjoy yourself also. Try to keep a good balance between school and home. It will make things easier for your family, and it will also help you keep your own sanity. If you are single without children, it may be a little easier for you to deal with this aspect. But that isn't to say that it won't be hard also. In some ways, it may be a little more difficult without that close support system. Be sure to have someone to lean on when things get tough, because they certainly will. Make sure you always have someone to talk to, whether it be friends, family, or classmates.

Not only do you need to find a balance between school and home, but you also need to find a balance between the clinical and didactic portions of your program. I think one of my biggest mistakes when I first started CRNA School was that I focused an enormous amount of my attention on the clinical aspects, largely overlooking much of the didactic portion. I was so nervous about looking stupid during a case, I would spend most of my time reading about techniques or studying topics I thought I might get pimped on. As my grades began to sink, I knew I had to find a different strategy. It's important to find some kind of balance between clinicals and classes. If you do great on your exams and have a 4.0 gpa, it will mean nothing if you can't get through clinicals. On the other hand, if you are doing great in the hospital, it also won't matter if your grades are suffering.

Try to find your sweet spot. I would lean towards spending more study time on didactics, but you have to decide for yourself what needs the most work at which time. I think that if you spend the proper study time in your classes, the clinical knowledge will just come by itself. It's impossible to know what a preceptor might ask you, and studying everything all at once is futile. Clinical technique will come with practice and persistence. Plus, performance reviews are subjective and you will often get the benefit of the doubt if you show that you are trying. Exams are very much objective and can't be interpreted to mean anything other than pass or fail. This is just my opinion, but one I wish I would have had from the start. It would have made things go much easier for me.

When it comes to deciding when to show up for clinicals, a general rule of thumb is to make sure your preceptor doesn't beat you there. It is going to show that you are interested and ready to work if you are already in the room by the time they get there. It would be even better if you had your set up done and you were ready to discuss the case. This might not always be possible, as some CRNA's get to work pretty early. As long as you get there in plenty of time to set up, talk to the patient, and go over the anesthetic plan, you shouldn't have any problems. When I first started CRNA School, I used to get to my clinical site at 5:30am for cases that didn't start until 7:30am. If that seems early, well...it's because it is. I wanted to make sure I had plenty of time to do everything I needed and study up if my case was unexpectedly changed. But I ended up spending a lot of time just sitting around after I had the room ready. As my program got further along, I started getting to the hospital at 6:00, 6:15, and eventually 6:30 in my last couple of semesters. The time you get there is completely up to you. Start out earlier than you think you need and see what works best. Usually no one will care what time you got there as long as you're ready to go.

While we are on the subject of working hours, we should discuss how you deal with the end of your shift also. Many programs will let you leave at the end of your scheduled shift, provided that there is someone else there to take care of the patient if you are still in a case. Sometimes, you might have to stay if there is no coverage. If you decide to stay and finish a case past your scheduled time on your own, this will be very much appreciated by your preceptor and the anesthesia gods will smile down upon you. However, I would recommend keeping this within reason. If the case should be finished within the next 30-60 minutes, then staying is probably the right choice. But if the case could go for another 5 hours, I don't think anyone would think less of you if you decided to leave. Use your own judgment and try to read your preceptor. Sometimes you can tell if they are expecting you to stay or if they don't care either way. If a preceptor insists on sending you home, don't fight it. If you really want to stay, ask politely if it would be ok if you finished the case. But if they keep telling you to go, then get the heck out of there.

Chapter Ten

Staying off the radar

As you go through anesthesia school, keep it a main goal of yours to stay out of the news, so to speak. Keep your head down and don't cause any waves. You don't want to be remembered for anything other than being a hard worker. Make sure they are aware that you know your stuff, but don't be a "know it all." If you disagree with someone, ask politely if they can explain their reasoning. Present your case and ask what they think. But don't argue with anyone or flat out tell them they are wrong about something. Even if you know without a shadow of a doubt that you are right, just let it go. Talk about it with your teachers and classmates for verification and move on. Try to go with the flow.

Remember that you are a guest and you have to play ball their way. Try not to get caught up in the gossip. Instead, just keep your eye on the prize. Worry about yourself and no one else. The last thing I'd mention about this has to do with politics and religion. Just like they don't belong at the dinner table, they don't belong in the OR (at least not as far as you're concerned). We all know how passionate people can be, so it would behoove you to keep such opinions to yourself.

Don't burn any bridges while you're in school, as it's always better to keep your options open. If you decide that you'd like to work for the anesthesia group at your clinical site, then of course you want to make a good name for yourself. But even if you want to work somewhere else, your reputation may travel right along with you. Many CRNAs and anesthesiologists know each other across the country. Just because you plan on living in another state doesn't mean your name won't follow you. Plus, someday you may want to come back. So don't get on anyone's bad side. Always keep your word and let them know you are there to do whatever is needed. Don't try to find the easy way out, always be available, and always look for new opportunities. Be honest and open and your good name will always stay with you no matter where you end up.

Chapter Eleven

Preparing for the Unexpected

As much as we would all like to prepare for our day before we go into the hospital, the cold hard truth is that we often have no idea what's coming our way until it's right in front of us. It's ok if you don't know the answer to something, as long as you know how to find the answers. Even as CRNA's, we often come across procedures or diseases that we haven't seen before. But we know where the resources are so we can be as informed as possible before a procedure starts. I think it is of vital importance to have some kind of electronic device that you can quickly find information on. If you're like many people, you probably already have a smart phone. If you do, then there are plenty of apps and web sites that have tons of information that can be accessed quickly. If you don't have a smart phone, I would recommend getting one before you start clinicals. I don't go a day without looking up a medication, a dose, or condition. The alternative to this is to carry several books around with you, something which may not even be allowed in the OR at your facility.

While I won't recommend any specific apps for your phone, I can tell you the different kinds you should probably have. Be sure to have a drug guide of some sort, preferably one specific to anesthesia. You should be able to quickly find a medication's dose, onset, duration, method of action, and administration instructions. It should tell you how to mix and administer commonly used drips. You also need quick access to surgical procedures and anesthetic implications for each. Another great help is to have a reference for specific disease states and how to manage them. I've seen some apps that cover each of the topics all in one place. Lastly, a simple search for things on the internet usually doesn't let me down. In fact, unless I'm looking up a drug, Google is usually my first stop to find information quickly. You can always ask another CRNA or anesthesiologist if you aren't familiar with something. I've been bailed out by my colleagues more times than I can count. Just remember, you don't necessarily have to know it all, but you have to know where to find it!

In the ICU or ER, you are usually surrounded by several other nurses who are there within seconds whenever an emergency arises. But in the operating room, you are in charge of dealing with emergencies until the anesthesiologist gets there. If your patient codes, you are the one calling the shots until then. It might take a few minutes for them to get there to take over, which is a long time when a patient isn't breathing or is in V-Fib. You absolutely have to know your BLS, ACLS, and PALS. In CRNA only groups, you will be the last stop, so it becomes even more important. In the ICU, this is something that might be easily forgotten (at least the details) since you can rely so heavily on other people. I know I let some things slip away in the time between my re-certifications. But in the OR, you have to act quickly and decisively. Don't forget that there are many more types of emergencies than the dreaded code. You need to know what to do in case of malignant hyperthermia, airway fires, laryngospasm, and bronchospasm, among other things. Know where the meds are and know where the carts are. Don't be afraid to call for help and know what you need to do in the first few minutes before that help gets there.

The other piece of advice I can give you is to try not to freak out when something bad or unexpected happens. It's always been said that CRNAs are paid so well because we are able to handle such situations. We're not making six figures because we can intubate someone and put some gas on. It's because of our ability to respond quickly in emergencies and unpredictable circumstances. As a CRNA, you must be able to adapt quickly. You can lose an airway or blood pressure in an instant. In one minute, you're waiting to roll back with your basic cystoscopy. In the next, that case is getting bumped for an emergency thoracotomy for a gunshot wound. You can prepare all day long, but anything can happen at any time. As Forrest Gump's momma would always say, anesthesia is like a box of chocolates...you never know what you're gonna get.

Chapter Twelve

The pre-op interview and post-op report

Before surgery, you are going to interview every patient unless it is an emergent case. The goal is to find out as much useful information as possible to help guide your anesthetic plan. First introduce yourself and confirm the patient's identity. Check their allergies and NPO status. Then go over the patient's medical and surgical history. If it helps, start at the head and work your way down the body. See if the patient or their family have ever had any complications related to anesthesia. Check their airway, looking at mallampati score, cervical range of motion, thyromental distance, neck size, and dentition. There may be a few more things your school or preceptor would also like for you to document in your airway examination. Make note of any missing, chipped, cracked, or loose teeth. Get a list of the patient's medications and make note of any anesthetic implications for each. As you do these exams more and more, it will get easier and faster. It may take you a while to go through each thing at first, but it will eventually become seamless and routine.

While you're in pre-op, make sure your patient has working IVs. If the case is complex or the patient has a cardiac history, an a-line may be required. If so, make sure it's in place before you go back to the operating room unless there is a reason to wait. Check all of the labs to make sure everything is normal or acceptable. If you think you might need blood during the case, make sure the patient is typed and crossed. Verify which antibiotics are ordered and know when they need to be re-dosed. Lastly, make sure your patient understands what is going to happen to them and what to expect. I usually explain that we will go back to the operating room and will have them move over to another bed. I tell them that I will hook up the monitors, put an oxygen mask over their face, and then call in the anesthesiologist to come in to help them go to sleep. Make sure they know when they will be going to sleep. If not, many patients will start to get nervous as you enter the operating room and move over to the bed. You will likely hear them say, "You know I'm not asleep yet, right?" It's vital to set expectations for every patient. You might have done this a hundred times, but they haven't and are curious about what's going to happen and when.

Once a case is complete, you will take your patient to the recovery room or ICU, making sure you have oxygen and medications if needed while transporting. When giving report to the receiving nurse, try to be short and to the point. They aren't looking for the patient's biography here. Give a brief medical history, including allergies and pertinent medications. List the amount of fluid given, blood lost, blood given, and urine output. Tell them which antibiotics were given, as well as any narcotics. You don't need to mention every anesthetic medication you administer. The nurse doesn't usually need to hear that you had the patient on Sevoflurane, that you gave 80mg of Lidocaine, or that you reversed the paralytic with Neostigmine and Robinul. They already assume you did all these things with most patients. Instead, just tell them the things you gave that were out of the ordinary. Of course, there will occasionally be a nurse that does want every detail and who asks a lot of questions. That is fine, but you typically don't need to waste your time giving this information. They usually don't want to hear it any more than you want to tell them.

Before you leave PACU, chart the vital signs and make sure the patient is stable. No one will fault you for spending a longer time in recovery to get them stabilized. If the patient's oxygen saturation is low, help the nurse get a nasal cannula, mask, or whatever is needed to fix the problem. If the blood pressure is too high or too low, then you need to get it back within an acceptable range before you leave. If the patient is having pain, please try to help alleviate it as much as you can. Although the nurse will have orders for pain medication, they will appreciate it greatly if you don't leave someone screaming in agony as you walk away. After all, pain relief is a major part of what we do, and it looks poorly on our profession when we don't get the job done. While you should try to get to your next case quickly, it shouldn't come at the cost of your patient's safety or comfort.

Chapter Thirteen

Working with others

You are going to be working with a lot more people than CRNAs and anesthesiologists. On a daily basis, you will be interacting with pre-op and PACU nurses, circulating nurses, surgical techs, anesthesia LPNs/techs, pharmacists...well you get the idea. These people can make your life much easier, but it will be more difficult for them if you don't get along. The best piece of advice I can give is to be nice! Make a good impression and try to be personable. Make sure you have a good attitude and be helpful when you can. You can't take care of any patient by yourself. You will need help getting supplies, positioning patients, getting meds, etc.

Of course, even if you're a jerk, you will still get the things you need. No one is going to sacrifice the well-being of a patient. But it might take a little longer to get non-emergency things, and they will likely not do it cheerfully. You will be able to feel the tension for sure. Anesthesia is hard enough. We need all the help we can get and we're happy to get it. I will say one more thing about Anesthesia LPNs/techs. If you are lucky enough to have them at your facility, treat them like gold. They are your lifeline, setting up in between cases, getting supplies, picking up meds, etc. I have not worked in a facility without them, and I can't imagine how much more stress that would cause.

Although it is important to be someone who is easy to get along with, you also don't want to be a pushover. Patient safety should always be your top priority. Don't let anyone rush you into making a poor decision. For example, there will be times when your patient will take a long time to wake up. There might be several people standing in the room waiting for you to extubate them so they can flip the room for the next case. The patient would probably be fine, but you just aren't quite comfortable yet. You will be tempted to pull the ET tube, thinking it's worth the gamble. Please don't do this. Don't do anything until you're ready. I'd rather have the turnover take a few minutes longer than the patient have to be re-intubated.

This doesn't just go for extubation of course. Don't ever start a case if you don't have everything you need to be safe. You might have those eyes on you again impatiently waiting. But do what you think is the safest thing. Also, don't ever let anyone move your patient without you taking care of the airway. Make sure everyone moves them on your count, with very few exceptions. These are just a few examples. You are going to experience many more of these types of issues every day. Just remember that patient safety is paramount. If you're not ready, then nothing should happen until you are.

Chapter Fourteen

Getting certified and finding a job

When school first starts, I'm sure the last thing you'll be thinking about is your Board Exam. Frankly, I don't blame you. You can't walk before you crawl, and you really should take things one day at a time. But keep the end game in the back of your mind as you move along. In other careers and in other classes, it's ok to take a test and then forget everything you studied. In anesthesia school, this type of thinking will surely come back to bite you. There is a lot of information that you won't be able to cram in 2 weeks before your certification exam.

Try to think of every lecture, every class, and every case as job training rather than school. It makes it much easier to remember things knowing that the information will help you be better in your profession. You're not just studying for a test...you're studying for a career. Once you've gotten about a year of school under your belt, it would probably be a good time to start gradually spending more time getting ready for the final showdown. Think about signing up for a review course like the one offered by Valley Anesthesia. They offer several comprehensive weekend courses throughout the year around the United States. You can also try a program like

Prodigy Anesthesia. They offer online exam simulation and tons of study material. Both of these options are pretty expensive, but they offer great preparation for boards and help tremendously with your confidence.

Unfortunately, I didn't have the funds for either of these programs. I was fortunate enough to get some old information from a previous student, but I procrastinated much longer than I should have. Although I passed the exam on the first try, I did not feel well prepared at all. I took the maximum amount of questions and I was sweating it out the entire way through. Don't do what I did. Focus mostly on your classes and your clinicals, but don't forget what is waiting at the end. Instead, make a plan and stick to it as much as you can. Try to answer 10 practice questions every day to start and go from there. If that proves to be too much, then make at least one day a week for it. Do what you can, but do it consistently. It will pay off in the long run!

It's hard to say at what point you should start looking for a job. Many employers won't hire you unless you're within 6 months of graduation. With that said, I'm sure there are several exceptions, particularly if you are looking to stay on at your current clinical site. The groups you have been working with know you pretty well after a fairly short period of time. Some may be willing to sign you during your first year.

However, I think most students usually find a job in that final 6 months. For my program, we graduated in May. Almost all of my class had a position lined up by February.

Try not to wait until the last minute to decide where you want to work. It can be a fairly easy process to find a job, or it can be very difficult. It's not that you won't be able to find work. Rather, it's more likely that there will be an overwhelming amount of positions available. If you know you want to work in a specific area, then the job hunt will come much easier for you. However, if you are open and willing to move anywhere, then it might take some time deciding the best fit for you. There are many types of jobs for CRNAs out there. You could work at a major trauma center or a more rural hospital. You could get a job at a GI center, surgery center, or pain clinic. Whatever you decide, try not to sign into a contract longer than a couple of years. You don't want to be stuck somewhere if you're miserable.

If you do sign a contract, read it carefully. Even better, have a lawyer read it. If there is something you don't agree with, propose changes and have them send another contract to you. While you have a long time to decide where you want to work, keep in mind that there is a credentialing process that a CRNA must go through for any place they want to work. This can sometimes take 3-4 months to get finalized before you can begin working. The sooner they can get started on it, the sooner you can start your career. Make sure you have enough money in the bank to cover that time without a paycheck or student loans.

Start your job search at one of the many sites offering this service specifically for anesthesia providers. Create a profile and build you resume. Include information that is related to the position of nurse anesthesia. Most employers won't care that you worked at a coffee shop for 3 years after high school. Be sure to document where you went to nursing school and where you worked as a registered nurse. Because nurse anesthesia is a profession in such high demand, many employers likely won't give your resume much thought. Just make it look professional, so they know you are someone who can be taken seriously. As long you passed an accredited CRNA program and got certified, they are usually more than happy to have you as an employee. Your grade point average and the quality of your papers probably won't even be considered. Keep this in mind as you go through your program and receive a grade less than you hoped for. In the end, everyone who makes it all the way through will be given the title of CRNA.

After you graduate, make sure you take a break before you begin working. You are going to deserve some time to yourself to decompress.

Try to go on vacation if you can. Either go before you take your board exam or wait until you've passed it to celebrate. I was dead broke when I graduated, so I just stayed at home. But I took the first week after school to just relax and spend time with my family. Then I hit the books hard and didn't stop until the exam. On the day of the exam, you should find out right after you submit your final answer whether or not you passed. Once you have that paper in your hand, feel free to tell the world how awesome you are...you've earned it!

Chapter Fifteen

Don't stop believing

I would love to tell you that reading this book is a guarantee of success, but the fact is that some people just aren't cut out for anesthesia. The same holds true for almost any profession. Sometimes all the determination in the world isn't enough to make a CRNA. It doesn't mean that the intelligence isn't there. It just means that they are meant to do something different. Some people find this out during the first or second semester on their own, so they decide to go back to nursing or do something else. Other times, this unfortunate reality must be presented in the form of bad grades or poor clinical evaluations. Nurse Anesthetists have their patients' lives in their hands. It's a great privilege that can't be simply given away...it must be earned. I hope you have what it takes to earn that privilege.

I know I don't have any golden tickets, but hopefully I have provided you with some valuable insight into the life of a CRNA student. I sometimes wish I could have blacked out much of what happened during my 28 months of training. But then I wouldn't be the CRNA I am today and I would have nothing to share with you. I made some great friends and learned a lot about myself. Don't be afraid to make your own mistakes, but try to learn as much as you can from the ones I made. 28-36 months probably seems like forever away. But you won't believe how fast it will go by. It's true that time flies when you're having fun. But it goes by even faster when you're too busy to realize that you're not having any fun at all. Keep your eye on the prize at the end of this long and arduous journey. Whenever you feel like quitting, just remember what you'll have if you choose to forge on. When that day comes, I'll be happy to call you my colleague.

CRNA MNEMONICS

120 TIPS, TRICKS, AND
MEMORY CUES TO HELP YOU
KICK-ASS IN CRNA SCHOOL

Introduction

Mnemonics can be a great tool to help your brain trigger specific information that you need to know quickly. This tactic can be used for exams, during questioning by instructors, or in your everyday clinical practice. It should be noted that memory tricks like these should not be thought of as a replacement for knowledge of the subject. You first need to understand the core concepts before the mnemonics will be able to help.

The good news is that once you have a grasp on the material you are trying to learn, mnemonics can make your life much easier. This is especially true in the world of anesthesia. There are thousands of diagnoses, labs, medications, symptoms, and treatments. Even after you learn something new, it is easy to get things mixed up.

For example, is there a greater risk of bleeding with a placenta accreta, increta, or percreta? What!? I feel your pain. Don't worry, this is covered later, along with tons of other difficult-to-remember anesthesia topics.

The idea here isn't to read this entire book to try to remember every single mnemonic. You'll drive yourself crazy that way. Rather, it is meant to be used as a guide as you progress through your anesthesia education and even as you begin your career as a provider.

When you start to cover a specific topic in school, come back to this book and see if there is a mnemonic for it. If you've graduated and there is something you just can't seem to remember, see if we have something that will help. This way, you will be learning as you go, and will be less likely to get the mnemonics mixed up.

Also, keep in mind that mnemonics will never have all the possible information for a specific topic. Only the most important things are covered, and sometimes items are left out for the sake of the mnemonic. It would be impossible to condense a 50-page chapter on the airway into a few words.

Some of these mnemonic devices are commonly known and I have used them myself many times. However, the majority of them are original creations by yours truly. Some of them may sound strange and funny. But this is a good thing! Those are the ones you are more likely to remember.

If something in this book just doesn't seem to be working for you, try to come up with your own mnemonic for that subject. It's not hard. Just try putting letters together to make up words or sentences that you can draw from when the time comes.

If you have any questions about anything in this book, please feel free to email me at contact@kickassnursing.com. Like us on Facebook, visit us on our web site at www.kickassnursing.com and check out the blog!

Airway

Epiglottitis – Symptoms

AIR RAID

Airway closed
Increased pulse
Restlessness

Retractions
Anxiety
Inspiratory stridor
Drooling

Epiglottitis can happen very quickly and is extremely dangerous. If not dealt with immediately, it could be life-threatening. As the epiglottis becomes more inflamed and irritated, it can swell to the point of completely blocking off the airway. The patient may lean forward to help air pass. They will often be drooling, have difficulty swallowing, stridor, hoarseness, and fever. They will be anxious and restless, especially as their airway closes more and more.

Epiglottitis – Treatment

NO FAITH

NPO
Oxygen

Fluids
Avoid examination of throat
Intubate
Tracheostomy
Humidification (cool mist)

Intubation is often the first treatment before the symptoms get worse. If the airway gets inflamed enough, it may be necessary to perform a tracheostomy. Antibiotics should be given once the airway is secure. Try not to examine the airway, as any stimulation can cause more inflammation. Give oxygen and fluids, and don't let them eat anything.

Larynx Cartilages

The **C**rocodile **E**ats **A**sian **C**orn **C**unningly

<u>9 Cartilages</u>

Thyroid
Cricoid
Epiglottis
Arytenoid (2)
Corniculate (2)
Cuneiform (2)

This should help you remember that the thyroid comes before the cricoid, meaning it is more superior. In between the thyroid and cricoid is the cricothyroid, a space you may want to familiarize yourself with. This is where you would perform a cricothyrotomy in a case of emergency.

Intrinsic Laryngeal Muscles - Function

Posterior **C**rico**A**rytenoids: Abduct vocal cords
Pulls **C**ords **A**part

Lateral **C**rico**A**rytenoids: Adduct vocal cords
Lures **C**ords **A**djacently

Crico**T**hyroids
Increase vocal **C**ord **T**ension

Thy**r**oarytenoids
Tranquilizes Cords (reduce cord tension)

The Posterior Cricoarytenoids are responsible for vocal cord abduction, which allows them to open. The Lateral Cricoarytenoids adduct the vocal cords, allowing them to close. The cricothyroids increase the vocal cord tension, while the thyroarytenoids relax the vocal cords. These both aid in changing tones during phonation.

Innervation of Larynx

[Motor]

R.E.M: **R**ecurrent and **E**xternal Superior for **M**otor

External **S**uperior Laryngeal: **C**ricothyroid Muscle

Recurrent Laryngeal: **A**ll other intrinsic muscles of larynx

SCAR: **S**uperior: **C**ricothyroid, **A**ll other: **R**ecurrent

Motor innervation of the larynx is taken care of by the Recurrent Laryngeal Nerve and the External Superior Laryngeal Nerve. The External Superior Laryngeal Nerve provides motor innervation of the cricothyroid muscle, while the Recurrent Laryngeal Nerve provides motor innervation to the rest of the intrinsic laryngeal muscles.

[Sensory]

SIR: **S**ensory supplied by **I**nternal Superior and **R**ecurrent

Internal **S**uperior Laryngeal: Vocal cords and **A**bove

Recurrent Laryngeal: **B**elow vocal cords

BRAS: **B**elow vocal cords: **R**ecurrent; **A**bove (and at) vocal cords: **S**uperior

Sensory innervation of the larynx is taken care of by the Internal Superior Laryngeal Nerve and the Recurrent Laryngeal Nerve. Motor innervation of the vocal cords and above is provided by the Internal Superior Laryngeal Nerve. Motor innervation below the vocal cords is provided by the Recurrent Laryngeal Nerve.

Predicting Difficult Airways: Mallampati Classification

Class I: Soft palate, tonsillar pillars, uvula
Class II: Tonsillar pillars and tip of uvula hidden by base of tongue
Class III: Soft palate visible only
Class IV: Soft palate not visible

PUSH

Pillars (I)
Uvula (II)
Soft Palate (III)
Hard palate (IV)

If you can see the soft palate, tonsillar pillars, and the uvula, your patient has a class I Mallampati. With class II, you will be able to see the base of the uvula, but the tonsillar pillars will be hidden. With a Mallampati III you will be able to see the soft palate, but not the pillars or uvula. In a class IV, the soft palate will be hidden also, allowing you to only see the hard palate.

Predicting Difficult Airways: LEMON Score

LEMON

Look Externally

Evaluate 3-3-2

Mallampati

Obstruction

Neck mobility

Look to see if there is something that could pose a problem physically, such as a foreign object or obvious deformity. Can the patient fit 3 fingers between the incisors, is the mandible length 3 fingers from the mentum to the hyoid, and is the distance from the hyoid to the thyroid at least 2 fingers (3-3-2)? Check the mallampati and look for an obstruction, such as a foreign object, tumor, or excessive soft tissue. Lastly, check to see how well the patient can move their head side to side and up and down.

Predicting Difficult Masking

<u>BONES</u>

<u>B</u>eard
<u>O</u>besity
<u>N</u>o teeth
<u>E</u>lderly
<u>S</u>nores

Masking a patient is going to be one of the most difficult things to learn and master in anesthesia. These predictors are not likely to help. A beard can create problems because it is difficult to create a seal around the hair. You will often find leaks of air in many places. With obesity, there is an abundance of soft tissue, impeding the airway. A patient with no teeth is sometimes difficult to mask because the structure in their mouth is lacking. Often, the mouth and all the soft tissue will fall onto itself, making it hard to get air passed. Elderly patients in general have decreased elasticity and range of motion. This stiffness can sometimes create a positioning problem while masking. Finally, snoring can often indicate sleep apnea, which indicates excess tissue blocking the airway while sleeping. This can make it difficult to get air in beyond the soft tissue.

Predicting Difficult Extraglottic Device Insertion

<u>RODS</u>

<u>R</u>estricted Mouth opening

<u>O</u>bstruction

<u>D</u>istorted or disrupted airway

<u>S</u>tuff lung, cervical Spine

Extraglottic airway devices are those that do not enter the trachea, but instead stay above the glottis. The most common example for this type of airway is the Laryngeal Mask Airway (LMA). Patients who have any restriction in the movement of their mouth or neck can cause difficulty in placing and/or ventilating through these devices. Obstructions in the airway, such as a tumor can also cause problems. In the same manner, a distorted airway or unusual anatomy can create the same types of difficulty.

Predicting Difficult Cricothyrotomy

<u>SHORT</u>

<u>S</u>urgery

<u>H</u>ematoma

<u>O</u>besity

<u>R</u>adiation distortion

<u>T</u>umor

A cricothyrotomy is an emergent procedure that can be used in cases of inability to ventilate or intubate. You'll find this spot in between the thyroid and cricoid cartilages. These may be more difficult to perform in patients who have had surgery in that region, or if there is a hematoma there. If a patient is obese, it can be difficult to find the correct area to enter. Radiation and tumors can also cause distortion in the neck and cricothyroid area, making it more difficult to penetrate and ventilate.

Laryngeal Mask Airway (LMA) Contraindications

HOODS

High pressures required

Obesity

Opioids required

Diabetics

Stomach full

A laryngeal mask airway (LMA) is a great tool that can be utilized in several scenarios instead of an endotracheal tube. However, sometimes it shouldn't be used. The main reason not to use it is because it doesn't protect against aspiration. In cases where aspiration risk is increased, an LMA should be avoided. This would be true with obesity, diabetics, and full stomachs. Additionally, when high pressures are needed during ventilation, the air could enter the stomach, increasing the risk. The same goes for a necessity for high dose opioids. These medications can increase nausea and slow gastric motility.

Nasotracheal Intubation Contraindications

CLIPS

Coagulopathy

Le Fort III fracture

Intranasal disease (severe – tumor, sinusitis)

Presence of CSF

Skull fracture (Basilar)

A nasotracheal intubation is not something that should be taken lightly. The structures you are passing by are very sensitive and the risk of damaging something is high. Because of the high vascularization of the area, patients who have a coagulopathy are at a much higher risk of bleeding. A Le Fort III fracture presents a problem because of the deformity and fractures of the nasal bones. Things like intranasal tumors and severe sinusitis could prevent the tube from passing and also cause trauma. The presence of CSF could indicate a skull fracture. Inserting a nasotracheal tube in this case increases the risk of penetrating into the cranial vault. Although this is extremely rare, avoid it if possible.

Aspiration Treatment

SPLAT

Suction
Positive pressure
Lavage
Antibiotics
Trendelenburg

If a patient aspirates, suction the mouth and endotracheal tube if present. Apply positive pressure to keep the alveoli open and prevent atelectasis. Put the patient in Trendelenburg position to promote the movement of any other substances away from the airway. Antibiotics will be needed to prevent and treat pneumonia. Bronchoscopy with lavage may be helpful also.

Diagnosing Poor Bilateral Breath Sounds after Intubation

DOPE

Displaced (right mainstem?)

Obstruction (kinked, bitten tube, mucous plug)

Pneumothorax

Esophagus

If the breath sounds are inadequate after intubation, the problem could be from multiple causes. If the breath sounds are diminished on the left, but adequate on the right, the tube might be in the right mainstem. Try pulling the tube back a little and rechecking. The patient may also have a pneumothorax. Check for other clinical signs indicating this. If the tube is in the esophagus, you will likely hear no breath sounds and you will see little to no end-tidal CO_2. If there is an obstruction, breath sounds will be diminished or absent also, and it will be extremely difficult to ventilate with high pressures. Check for possible sources, such as a kinked tube, biting, or mucous plug.

To Get a Better View During Laryngoscopy

BURP

Backwards

Upwards

Right

Posterior

This is the position pressure should be placed to get a better view of the vocal cords. After getting the blade into a good position in the mouth, use your right hand to perform this maneuver. Then direct someone else to do the same maneuver if it helps bring a better look at the cords into view.

Rapid Sequence Induction

The Seven Ps

Preparation
Pre-oxygenation
Pre-treatment
Paralysis
Protection and Positioning
Placement (with proof)
Post-intubation management

Rapid sequence intubations are done for a variety of reasons, including trauma, full stomach, risk for aspiration, etc. To do it right, make sure you prepare in advance. Properly pre-oxygenate, since you will want to avoid ventilating after the medications are given. If using Anectine, consider pre-treating with a non-depolarizer, such as rocuronium, to decrease fasciculations. Place the patient in optimal position for intubation and protect the airway by having someone hold pressure on the cricoid cartilage. Once they are paralyzed, intubate quickly and verify placement. After placement is verified and the cuff is inflated, pressure can be released from the cricoid.

Cardiovascular
System

Adrenergic Receptors

<u>Beta-1</u> affects the Heart (**1 Heart**)

<u>Beta-2</u> affects the Lungs (**2 Lungs**)

Alpha-agonist Potency: <u>E</u>pinephrine > <u>N</u>orepinephrine > <u>D</u>opamine > <u>I</u>soproterenol

<u>E</u>very <u>N</u>udist <u>D</u>emands <u>I</u>nclusion

Beta-agonist Potency: <u>I</u>soproterenol > <u>E</u>pinephrine > <u>N</u>orepinephrine > <u>D</u>opamine

<u>I</u> <u>E</u>at <u>N</u>utty <u>D</u>onuts

Keep in mind that each of these is a generalization, and not always the rule. For example, Beta 1 receptors are mostly found on the heart and beta 2 mostly in the lungs. But they are also in many other areas of the body and affect more than just the heart and lungs. In general, at the alpha receptors, epinephrine is more potent than norepinephrine, which is more potent than dopamine and isoproterenol. But the same order may not hold true at each specific alpha-1 and alpha-2 receptors.

Pacemaker Codes

PaSeR

Pa – Chamber **Pa**ced
Se – Chamber **Se**nsed
R – **R**esponse to sensing

First Letter – Chamber Paced
Second Letter – Chamber Sensed
Third Letter – Response to Sensing

Example: VVI = Ventricular Paced, Ventricular Sensed, Inhibited Mode

Coronary Blood Supply

Anterior wall supplied by **LAD**
Changes seen in leads V1-V4

Lateral wall supplied by **LAD** or **O**btuse
Marginal
Seen in I, avl, V5, V6

Inferior wall supplied by **RCA**
Seen in Leads II, III, avf

Posterior wall supplied by **PDA**
Seen as depression in V1, and V2

The **Ant** is fed by the **LAD** in the morning
If it's **Late**, it is fed by the **LAD** or the **O**ld **M**an
From this, you can **Infer** that these **R**ations
Cause **A**rguments
I have a **Poster** that shows **P**ublic **D**isplays of
Affection

Even I'll admit this mnemonic is pretty silly. But I
was having a heck of a time remembering the
blood supply, so I came up with this little story
about an ant and how it gets food every day.
Also, I threw in some random comment about a
poster. It hasn't failed me yet, but I'm all ears if
you have come across a better one!

Catecholamine synthesis

This is a tough one, but hopefully this mnemonic will help you bring it all together. First, let's review the basic conversion of L-Tyrosine all the way to epinephrine:

L-tyrosine is converted to L-Dopa by Tyrosine Hydroxylase.
L-Dopa is converted to Dopamine by Dopa Decarboxylase.
Dopamine is converted to Norepinephrine by Dopamine B-Hydroxylase.
Norepinephrine is converted to Epinephrine by Phenylethanolamine n-methyltransferase.

L-Tyrosine (Tyrosine Hydroxylase – **TH**) -> **L-D**opa (Dopa Decarboxylase – **DD**) -> **D**opa**mine** (Dopamine B-Hydroxylase – **DBH**) -> **No**repinephrine (phenylethanolamine n-methyltransferase – **PNMT**) -> **Ep**inephrine

Little **T**igger, on **Th**ursday, met **L**ittle **D**opey

Little **D**opey took **D**unkin **D**onuts to the **D**iamond**Mine**

The **D**iamond**Mine** was **D**esigned **B**y **H**umans in **No**vember

That **No**vember, **P**oor **N**ew **M**exico **T**eens visited **Ep**cot

Pre-Bypass Checklist

An **A**pple **C**an **I**ncrease **M**yocardial **P**rotection

Anticoagulation

Anesthesia

Cannulation

IVs

Monitors

Pupils

Terminating Bypass

CVP (6 **C**s, 4 **V**s, 6 **P**s)

Cold
Conduction
Coagulation
Cardiac Output
Calcium
Cells

Ventilation
Vaporizer
Visualize
Volume

Predictions
Pressure
Pressor
Protamine
Potassium
Pacer

Nervous System

Cranial Nerves

<u>O</u>h <u>O</u>h <u>O</u>h <u>T</u>o <u>T</u>ouch <u>A</u>nd <u>F</u>eel <u>A</u> <u>G</u>irl's <u>V</u>agina <u>A</u>nd <u>H</u>einie

I.   <u>O</u>lfactory
II.   <u>O</u>ptic
III. <u>O</u>culomotor
IV.   <u>T</u>rochlear
V.   <u>T</u>rigeminal
VI.   <u>A</u>bducens
VII. <u>F</u>acial
VIII. <u>A</u>coustic (vestibulocochlear)
IX.   <u>G</u>lossopharyngeal
X.   <u>V</u>agus
XI.   <u>A</u>ccessory (spinal)
XII. <u>H</u>ypoglossal

There are several variations to this mnemonic, but this one has served me best throughout the years. Make sure you know the functions of each of these nerves and how to perform a neurological examination to test how well they are working.

Cranial Nerves - Motor, Sensory, or Both?

Some **S**ay **M**arry **M**oney, **B**ut **M**y **B**rother **S**ays **B**ig **B**oobs **M**atter **M**ost

I.   **S**ensory
II.   **S**ensory
III. **M**otor
IV.   **M**otor
V.   **B**oth
VI.   **M**otor
VII. **B**oth
VIII. **S**ensory
IX.   **B**oth
X.   **B**oth
XI.   **M**otor
XII. **M**otor

Each cranial nerve has either a motor function, sensory function, or a mixture of the two. For example, the olfactory nerve (I) has the main sensory function of smell. The oculomotor nerve (III) has the main motor function of eye movement.

101

Nerve Damage: Lithotomy Position

FOPPS

Femoral Nerve
Obturator Nerve
Peroneal (Common) Nerve
Saphenous Nerve
Sciatic Nerve

The femoral nerve is commonly damaged when stretched by excessive angulation of the thigh in lithotomy position. The obturator nerve can get stretched by excessive flexion of the thigh to the groin. The common peroneal nerve may get damaged by compression of the lateral aspect of the legs at the head of the fibula against the stirrup supports. The saphenous nerve could be affected with compression of the medial aspect of the legs against the stirrup supports. Finally, the sciatic nerve may be stretched by excessive external rotation of the leg when placing the patient into lithotomy position

Neurotransmitters

[Excitatory]

Great **DANES**

Glutamic acid
Dopamine
Acetylcholine, **A**spartic acid
Norepinephrine
Epinephrine
Serotonin

[Inhibitory]

Gleeful **Ga**ngsters

Glycine
GABA

Somatic vs Autonomic Nervous System

Som**a**tic
Controls **S**keletal **M**uscle (**S**tarted **M**anually)

Autonomic
Sympathetic and Parasympathetic (**Auto**matic)

Parasympathetic
Sedentary functions (**Pa**ssive)

Sympathetic
Fight or Flight (**S**peeding)

The Somatic Nervous System controls the skeletal muscles. This system is under voluntary control. This means that we move it when we want to move it. The autonomic system is involuntary and involves the parasympathetic and sympathetic systems. Our fight or flight response involves the sympathetic nervous system, while many sedentary, passive functions are taken care of by the parasympathetic nervous system.

Nerve Fibers - Order of Blockade

Nerve fibers A, B, C

1st: **B**
2nd: **C**, **A**-**d**elta
3rd: **A**-**g**amma
4th: **A**-**b**eta
5th: **A**-**a**lpha

1st: **B**est
2nd: **C**ats **A**nd **D**ogs
3rd-5th: **AAA**'s **G**et **B**lood **A**lways

When local anesthetic is injected into nerves, there is an order by which they are blocked and unblocked. The fibers blocked first are the B fibers, followed by the C fibers and A-delta fibers. The rest of the A fibers are blocked after that, starting with A-gamma, then A-beta, and finally A-alpha. When the anesthetic wears off, this happens in reverse, so that the A-alpha fibers are unblocked first, and the B fibers are unblocked last.

Oculocardiac reflex

Five and dime

The oculocardiac reflex happens when traction is placed on the extraocular muscles or when the eyeball gets compressed. This is because there is a connection between the Trigeminal (V) nerve and the Vagus (X) nerve. This is where Five (V) and Dime (X) comes from. When this reflex gets triggered, you may see bradycardia, and may even progress to asystole. The trigger should be immediately stopped or removed. You can give Robinul or Atropine to treat it as necessary.

Methods to Reduce ICP

MADE

Mannitol

Avoid anxiety, coughing, etc.

Decrease PaCO2

Elevate HOB

Intracranial pressure (ICP) can be reduced by using Mannitol, as it is an osmotic diuretic. Elevating the head of the patient's bed may also help by draining cerebral blood and CSF. If you decrease the PaCO2, it will cause cerebral arterial vasoconstriction, thereby reducing the ICP. Any kind of action that will increase the blood pressure will also likely cause an increase in ICP. Because of this, it is wise to avoid anything that may cause coughing, anxiety, straining, etc.

Spinal Cord Blood Supply

1 Anterior Spinal Artery (supplies the anterior **2/3**)

3-2=1

2 Posterior Spinal Arteries (supplies the posterior **1/3**)

3-1=2

Artery of **A**damkiewicz: major blood supplier of **A**nterior Spinal Artery

AAA

The anterior two-thirds of the spinal cord is supplied by the anterior spinal artery. The posterior two-thirds of the spinal cord is supplied by the 2 posterior spinal arteries. The major supply to the anterior spinal artery is the Artery of Adamkiewicz. This artery shows up often on tests, so keep it in mind. When this particular artery is damaged, that blood supply to the anterior spinal artery is greatly diminished, and can cause anterior spinal artery syndrome. You could see incontinence, and paralysis to some degree of the lower extremities.

C5 to T1 Nerve Branches (Lateral to Medial)

MARMU

Musculocutaneous

Axillary

Radial

Median

Ulnar

As part of the brachial plexus, these nerve branches are important to know and understand. They provide motor and sensory innervation to the almost the entire upper limb. Damage to the brachial plexus can often happen from excessive stretching or compression.

Brachial Plexus Segments

Randy **T**ravis **D**rinks **C**old **B**eer

Roots

Trunks

Divisions

Cords

Branches

The brachial plexus consists of five roots, three trunks, six divisions, three cords, and five branches. The roots are the five anterior rami of the spinal nerves. These roots then go into the 3 trunks (superior, middle, and inferior). The six divisions include 3 anterior and 3 posterior from the superior, middle, and inferior trunks. From there, we have the cords, which include the posterior, lateral, and medial. After that, the branches are the musculocutaneous, axillary, radial, median, and ulnar nerves.

Layers of the Scalp

SCALP

Subcutaneous

Connective tissue

Aponeurosis

Loose connective tissue

Pericranium

It may be helpful to know which layers the neurosurgeon is going through before getting to the brain during a craniotomy. But aside from this, I can't imagine much of a use for this information to an anesthesia provider. However, it has come up in testing many times, so keep it with you for future reference.

CSF Flow from the Choroid Plexus

Love My 3 Silly 4-Legged Mammoths

Lateral Ventricle

Monroe (Foramina of)

3rd Ventricle

Sylvian Aqueduct

4th Ventricle

Luschka (Foramina of)

Magendie (Foramen of)

Respiratory System

Alkalosis vs Acidosis

ROME

Respiratory – **O**pposite
Metabolic – **E**qual

-If the alkalosis is due to a Respiratory cause, pH will be high and pCO2 will be low
-If the acidosis is due to a Respiratory cause, pH will be low and pCO2 will be high
(Opposite)

-If the alkalosis is due to a Metabolic cause, pH and HCO3 will be high
-If the acidosis is due to a Metabolic cause, pH and HCO3 will be low
(Equal)

Henderson-Hasselbalch Equation

<u>HK</u> + **<u>AHA</u>**

Or

<u>H</u>ong <u>K</u>ong + <u>A</u>merican <u>H</u>ospital <u>A</u>ssociation

p**<u>H</u>** = p**<u>K</u>**a + $\log_{10}$(**<u>A</u>**⁻/**<u>HA</u>**)

The complexities of the Henderson-Hasselbalch equation is beyond the scope of this book. However, this quick little mnemonic can hopefully help you to remember the foundation of it.

Asthma – Treatment

ASTHMA

Adrenergics (B2 agonists – e.g. Albuterol)
Steroids
Theophylline
Hydration
Mask (oxygen)
Antibiotics, **A**nticholinergics

When thinking about treatments for asthma, consider whether or not it is an acute attack. When dealing with an asthma attack, the first choice is usually an albuterol inhaler. Before going back to the operating room, you may want to think about a prophylactic breathing treatment. If you are in a case and the patient has a bronchospasm, there are a couple things you can try. First, give some albuterol. In most facilities, if a patient is intubated, you can simply place the inhaler in a 60 cc syringe, and attach the syringe to the top of the ET tube (where the CO_2 line connects). If that doesn't work, racemic epinephrine may be necessary. If that doesn't work or you don't have much time, you may just need to give epinephrine through the IV.

Lung Volumes

Tidal Volume (TV):
Amount of gas in a Typical Ventilation (normal breath)

Inspiratory Reserve Volume (IRV):
Inspiration Remaining Volume (after a normal inspiration)

Expiratory Reserve Volume (ERV):
Expiration Remaining Volume (after a normal expiration)

Residual Volume (RV):
Remaining Volume (after maximal expiration)

Tidal Volume (TV) is the amount of gas inspired or expired with each normal breath. Inspiratory Reserve Volume (IRV) is the maximum amount of additional air that can be inspired at the end of a normal inspiration. Expiratory Reserve Volume (ERV) is the maximum volume of additional air that can be expired at the end of a normal expiration. Residual Volume (RV) is the volume of air remaining in the lung after a maximal expiration. This is the only lung volume which cannot be measured with a spirometer.

Oxyhemoglobin Dissociation Curve

CADET

$\underline{C}$O2

$\underline{A}$cid

2,3-$\underline{D}$PG (now recognized by many as 2,3-BPG)

$\underline{E}$xercise

$\underline{T}$emperature

Mo$\underline{R}$e of each: $\underline{R}$ight shift

$\underline{L}$ess of each: $\underline{L}$eft shift

When a shift to the right occurs, it means that oxygen has a decreased affinity for hemoglobin. This means that hemoglobin will have a harder time binding to oxygen, but that the oxygen it does have can be released easier to the tissues. When you exercise, your body's tissues need more oxygen, which is why the curve shifts right during this time. The same thing happens when there is an increased CO2, hyperthermia, increased 2,3-DPG, and in acidotic conditions.

When a shift to the left occurs, it means oxygen has an increased affinity for hemoglobin. Because of this, hemoglobin will have a harder time releasing the oxygen to the tissues. This happens when CO2 is decreased, during alkalosis, during relaxation, hypothermia, and with a decreased 2,3-DPG.

Factors that Decrease FRC

PANGOS

Pregnancy
Ascites
Neonate
GETA
Obesity
Supine position

Functional Residual Capacity (FRC) is the amount of air that is still in the lungs at the end of a normal expiration. When there is anything present that causes more resistance for the lungs to expand, FRC will be lower. For example, when laying in the supine position, there is more weight coming down on the lungs and diaphragm. Also, the abdominal contents move cephalad, further displacing the diaphragm. The same thing holds true for pregnancy, ascites, and obesity because of the limited room for expansion. In neonates, the outward recoil of the chest wall is decreased, thereby decreasing the FRC. During general anesthesia, the thoracic muscles are relaxed, which allows more movement of the abdominal contents against the diaphragm.

Pediatrics/
Obstetrics

Fetal Accelerations/Decelerations

VEAL CHOP

Variable Decelerations – **C**ord Compression
Early Decelerations – **H**ead Compression
Accelerations – **O**kay!
Late Decelerations – **P**lacental Insufficiency

Alternative...

Very **D**irty **C**hildren
Variable **D**ecelerations – **C**ord Compression

Every **D**ay **H**ero
Early **D**ecelerations – **H**ead Compression

Lucky **D**og **P**aws
Late **D**ecelerations – **P**lacental Insufficiency

Fetal Non-Stress Test

Non-reactive

Non-stress test

is

Not good!

It almost sounds counter-intuitive, but it makes sense if you know what it's testing for. If a fetus has a reaction during a non-stress test, it means all is well. They are moving and reacting appropriately. On the other hand, if the fetus does not react during a non-stress test, it could indicate a very serious problem.

Preeclampsia – Medications

My **L**oving **B**aby **H**as **D**emands

Magnesium

Labetalol

Betamethasone

Hydralazine

Dexamethasone

Hydralazine and Labetalol will help to bring the blood pressure under control. The steroids will help to speed up the fetal lung maturity in case she is born early. Dexamethasone may also help to slow the progression of preeclampsia. Magnesium is sometimes given to help prevent seizures. The only cure for preeclampsia is delivery of the baby. If the symptoms are bad enough, delivery will be forced to solve the problem.

Severe Pre-Eclampsia - Symptoms

HELLP

Hemolysis
Elevated **L**iver enzymes
Low **P**latelet count

Alternative...

TRIPLE

Thrombocytopenia

Renal Insufficiency

Intracranial disturbance

Proteinuria, **P**ressure (BP) is high

LFT Elevation

Edema

When does Pre-eclampsia become Eclampsia?
Here's a rhyme to help you remember:

If the patient has seizures and you agree
It's now Eclampsia (drop the "pre")

Congenital Cyanotic Heart Defects

One big **trunk** (**Trunc**us Arteriosus)

Two interchanged vessels (Transposition of the Great Vessels)

Three: **Tri**cuspid Atresia

Four: **Tetra**logy of Fallot

Five words: Total Anomalous Pulmonary Venous Return

Alternative...

5 T's

Truncus Arteriosus
Transposition of the Great Vessels
Tricuspid Atresia
Tetralogy of Fallot
Total Anomalous Pulmonary Venous Return

Obtaining Obstetric History

GTPAL

Gravida

Term pregnancies

Premature births

Abortions

Live births

When taking care of a pregnant patient, you still must perform a regular history and physical like you would with any other patient. But you should also find out relevant information regarding their obstetric history. Determine how many pregnancies they've had, how many went to term, how many were born premature, and how many abortions and live births they have had. This type of information can help you calculate risks for problems that may arise while they're in your care.

Obstetric Definitions

Gravida: Number of Pre**G**nancies

Nulligravida: **N**ever been pregnant

Multigravida: **Multi**ple pregnancies (at least 2)

Primigravida: **Primi**ng the uterus (First pregnancy)

Parity: Number of births with **P**ossibility (viable)

Nullipara: **N**ever given live birth

Multipara: **Multi**ple live births (at least 2)

Primipara: **Prim**ed Uterus (one live birth)

Here's an example: a patient who is a gravida 5, para 4 has had 5 pregnancies and 4 of those pregnancies led to a live birth. The 5th may be her current pregnancy, or one that was aborted (voluntary or otherwise). She would be considered multigravida and multipara.

Fetal Stations

FISHING

-3: **F**loating high

-2: **I**n the right direction

-1: **S**ettling in

0: **H**alfway there

+1: **I**nching out

+2: **N**early there

+3: **G**et the crown

The fetal station is referring to where the presenting part of the fetus is in the mother's pelvis. The ideal presenting part is the head, but it can be whichever body part is in the canal. At +3, crowning should begin and delivery is imminent.

Placental Abnormalities

Accreta, **I**ncreta, **P**ercreta

A comes before **I** comes before **P**

It gets worse the further you go in the alphabet

A < I < P

In placenta accreta, the placenta attaches to the myometrium. With placenta increta, the placenta invades into the myometrium. A placenta percreta will invade past the myometrium and through the outer layer of the uterus. It can then attach to other organs outside the uterus, such as the bladder or rectum. Each abnormality increases the risk for bleeding, but percreta poses a much higher threat than accreta.

Prevention of Pre-Term Labor - Tocolytics

It's **N**ot **M**y **T**ime

Indomethacin (NSAIDs)

Nifedipine (Ca channel blocker)

Magnesium sulfate

Terbutaline (Beta Agonist)

Or

MINT

Magnesium Sulfate

Indomethacin (NSAIDs)

Nifedipine (Ca Channel Blocker)

Terbutaline (Beta Agonist)

Obstetrical Hemorrhage – Causes

(Antepartum hemorrhage)

Ante**P**artum

Abruption (of placenta)
Previa (placenta)

(Intrapartum hemorrhage)

URAP

Uterine **R**upture
Abnormal **P**lacentation

(Postpartum hemorrhage)

4 T's
Thrombin
Tissue
Tone
Trauma

Aspiration Risk Factors in Pregnancy

DRIP

Delayed gastric emptying

Relaxed gastroesophageal sphincter (due to circulating progesterone)

Increased intragastric **P**ressure

When it comes to airway management in the pregnant population, aspiration is one of the greatest risks. There is some debate as to when you should treat a pregnant patient as though they had a full stomach, but after 8-12 weeks might be a good rule of thumb. After delivery, they should still be considered a full stomach up to 6 weeks postpartum.

Drugs That Don't Cross the Placenta

SIGN Him

Succinylcholine

Insulin

Glycopyrrolate

Non-Depolarizing neuromuscular blockers

Heparin

There are several factors that affect the transfer of drugs across the placenta. This includes the drug's molecular weight, its protein binding, lipid solubility, and unionization. All paralytics, heparin, insulin, and glycopyrrolate will not cross the placenta. Therefore, they are safe to give to the mother with little regard to the fetus.

Factors that Affect Placental Transfer

PLUM

Protein Binding

Lipid Solubility

Unionization

Molecular weight

It's important to know which medications cross the placenta and why. Sometimes, it may not matter much if the fetus gets the medication also. But it is typically something you'll want to take into consideration. Medications that have more protein binding are less likely to cross the placenta. The same holds true for those which have a high lipid solubility, high molecular weight, and those which more ionized.

Coagulation
and Bleeding
Disorders

Hemophilia – Differentiating between A, B, and C

Hemophilia A: Factor VIII Deficiency
A: **Ate** (8)

Hemophilia B: Factor IX Deficiency (Christmas Disease)
B: I **B**elieved in **Santa** at **9** years old (9)

Hemophilia C: Factor XI Deficiency
C: **Ca**l**l** me (11)

Hemophilia A is a deficiency of Factor VIII (8), which can be remembered by the word "Ate." Hemophilia B is a deficiency of Factor IX (9), also known as Christmas Disease. Just think back to when you were 9, you "Believed (B) in Santa (Christmas)." Hemophilia C is a deficiency of Factor XI (11). The word "Call" has a C and and 11 (using the L's as 11).

Coagulation Factors

Foolish **P**eople **T**ry **C**limbing **L**ong **S**lopes **A**fter **C**hristmas...**S**ome **P**eople **H**ave **F**allen

I.	**F**ibrinogen
II.	**P**rothrombin
III.	**T**issue Thromboplastin
IV.	**C**alcium
V.	**L**abile Factor
VII.	**S**table Factor
VIII.	**A**ntihemophilic Factor
IX.	**C**hristmas Factor
X.	**S**tuart-Prower Factor
XI.	**P**TA
XII.	**H**ageman Factor
XIII.	**F**ibrin Stabilizing Factor

Factor VI is Accelerin, but plays no role in blood coagulation

Vitamin K Dependent Clotting Factors

SEVEral **TEN**d **TO(2)** **Ni**cely **S**top **C**lots

II (Two)

VII (Seven)

IX (Nine)

X (Ten)

Protein S

Protein C

Or

1972

X (**1**0)

IX (**9**)

VII (**7**)

II (**2**)

Medications

Antidotes

Coumadin – Vitamin K
Cold Vampire

Heparin – Protamine Sulfate
Hot Pepper

Benzodiazepines – Romazicon (Flumazenil)
Banana Republic

Opiates – Naloxone (Narcan)
Old Navy

Tylenol – Mucomyst
Time Magazine

Beta Blockers – Glucagon
Bradycardia's Gone

Barbiturates

Every **G**irl

Deserves **R**oses

Enhance **G**ABA

Depress the **R**AS

GABA (gamma aminobutyric acid) is an important inhibitory neurotransmitter in the brain, a substance that many anesthetics capitalize on. By enhancing GABA, barbiturates increase the level of inhibition. The RAS (reticular activating system) functions to maintain wakefulness. By depressing this, barbiturates are able to cause patients to sleep.

Common barbiturates:

Thiopental, Methohexital (Brevital)

Neuromuscular Blockers (Non-Depolarizing): Long-Acting

My **G**irl **P**atty **P**acks **D**ouble **D**'s

Metocurine

Gallamine

Pancuronium

Pipecuronium

Doxacurium

d-tubocurarine

These are all long-acting non-depolarizing neuromuscular blockers, though you may only see Pancuronium used in your practice today. However, it's still a good idea to have them memorized as you may still see some of them show up on testing.

Neuromuscular Blockers (Non-Depolarizing): Intermediate-Acting

CRAVE

Cisatracurium

Rocuronium

Atracurium

Vecuronium

All of the intermediate-acting non-depolarizing neuromuscular blockers are still in use today. Rocuronium can be used for rapid sequence intubations if necessary. These medications generally last from 30 – 90 minutes.

Neuromuscular Blockers (Non-Depolarizing): Short-Acting

Mivacurium is **M**omentary

Long-acting neuromuscular blockers have a duration of action longer than 40 minutes. Intermediate-acting typically last in the 30-40 minute range. Mivacurium can last 12-20 minutes.

NMB Reversal Agents (with Corresponding Anti-Cholinergic)

Neosti**g**mine – **G**lycopyrrolate

Pyridosti**g**mine – **G**lycopyrrolate

Ed**rop**honium – At**rop**ine

Sugammadex – Flying **S**olo

The most commonly used reversal agents are neostigmine and now Sugammadex, but you may want to learn the other 2 just in case you see it on a test. All are anti-cholinesterases, with the exception of Sugammadex, which is why an anti-cholinergic is not needed when you give it.

Propofol (Diprivan)

SHARP LAD

Stimulates GABA
Hypotension
Antiemetic qualities
Respiratory depression
Pain on injection

Lipid soluble
Avoid in allergies (soybean oil, glycerol, egg lecithin)
Decreases CBF and ICP

Propofol is a great medication that can be used versatilely in the field of anesthesia. It is used for entire cases under MAC, such as endoscopy, port placements, and other short cases with minimal stimulation. It is often used during induction for general anesthesia cases, and it is used in combination with other drugs during TIVA cases. It has a rapid onset and is short acting. Watch for hypotension and respiratory depression. It can also cause a lot of pain at the injection site, so is often preceded by IV Lidocaine.

Ketamine (Ketalar)

SUPER BRAINS

Stimulates SNS
Urinary Excretion
Phencyclidine (PCP) derivative
Emergence delirium
Respiratory depression minimal

Bronchodilator
Recreational abuse
Analgesia
Increased BP, HR, CO, ICP, CVP, PAP, CI
NMDA receptor antagonist
Salivation

Ketamine is a phencyclidine (PCP) derivative that works well to provide analgesia and dissociation, while keeping the respiratory system intact for the most part. It does stimulate the sympathetic nervous system, so you will often see an increase in heart rate and blood pressure. It is not recommended if there is a desire to keep ICP low. It causes salivation, so can be used with an anticholinergic, such as glycopyrrolate to help. It has a high abuse potential, and is widely used recreationally because of this.

Etomidate (Amidate)

HAMPERS

Hypnotic
Adrenocortical suppression (long-term use)
Minimal CV effects
Pain on injection (mixed in propylene glycol)
Esterases (and hepatic metabolism)
Respiratory depression
Seizure activity (myoclonic movements)

A common use for etomidate is as a replacement for Propofol in patients with cardiac disease. Propofol can cause severe cardiovascular depression, something very minimal with etomidate. Long term use may lead to adrenocortical suppression, and there have been instances of seizure activity. As with Propofol, it does cause pain at the injection site. To attenuate this, IV Lidocaine prior to injection would be helpful.

Dexmedetomidine (Precedex)

AB RASH

Alpha-2 agonist
Bradycardia

Respiratory depression mild
Analgesia, anxiolysis
Sedation
Hypotension

Precedex is similar to Clonidine, in that it is an alpha-2 agonist. As with Clonidine, it will cause hypotension and sedation. It also provides excellent pain relief, while keeping the respiratory depression very minimal. Bradycardia should be expected and monitored closely.

Succinylcholine (Anectine)

<u>MD PHOBIA</u>

<u>M</u>alignant Hyperthermia trigger
<u>D</u>epolarizing neuromuscular blocker

<u>P</u>seudocholinesterase metabolism
<u>H</u>yperkalemia, Histamine release (minimal)
<u>O</u>verdose = Phase II block
<u>B</u>radycardia (due to muscarinic stimulation)
<u>I</u>ncreases IOP, ICP, intragastric pressure
<u>A</u>cetylcholine mimicker

Succinylcholine is the only depolarizing neuromuscular blocker used clinically. It is also the only one that is capable of triggering malignant hyperthermia. It is metabolized by pseudocholinesterase, so patients with a deficiency of this will have a much longer time to wait before it wears off. It is known to cause an increase in ICP, IOP, and intragastric pressure, so it should be avoided in patients where this would be detrimental. Because of its muscarinic stimulation, it can cause bradycardia, something that can be extreme in repeated dosing.

Pitocin (Oxytocin)

[Side Effects]

PITOCIN

Pressure is elevated
Intake and Output
Tetanic Contractions
Oxygen decrease in fetus
Cardiac arrhythmia
Irregular fetal heart beat
Nausea and Vomiting

[Uses]

AID

After Suction D&C
Induction of labor
Decrease postpartum uterine bleeding

Pitocin is great at causing the uterus to contract, so it is often used to start the induction of labor. It is used for the same reason after labor, c-section, or dilation and curettage. In the postpartum period, the uterus must contract to prevent or stop any bleeding. This medication is absolutely contraindicated in pregnant women who are not ready to induce labor.

Methergine (Methlyergonovine)

BASIC

Blood pressure increases

Alpha stimulation (causes arterial vasoconstriction)

Semisynthetic ergot alkaloid

Increases tone, rate and amplitude of contraction

Contraindicated in severe hypertension, PIH and cardiac disease

Methergine is most commonly used in anesthesia to help with postpartum bleeding. When Pitocin isn't enough to get the uterus to contract, this drug can be helpful by increasing the uterine tone, rate, and amplitude or its contraction. It should be avoided in patients with severe hypertension and cardiac disease, as it can cause extreme increases in blood pressure.

Hemabate (Carboprost)

STADIUM

Synthetic analogue of prostaglandin F2

Temperature increases

Airway constriction and wheezing

Diarrhea

Increases CO, BP and PVR

Uterine contraction stimulated

Myometrial calcium increases

Hemabate is most often used in anesthesia to help stop postpartum bleeding. As with Methergine, it is usually a back-up plan when Pitocin doesn't do the trick. It stimulates uterine contraction and increases myometrial calcium. It can cause airway constriction, so is contraindicated in asthmatics unless it's an emergency. The patient's core body temperature can increase as well.

Misoprostol (Cytotec)

Mis O Pro Stol

Miscarriage (induce labor or induce abortion)

Open PDA (Al**pro**stadil – synthetic PGE1)

Protects **Sto**mach (against NSAIDs)

Misoprostol can be used orally, sublingually, buccally, intravaginally, or rectally. It may be used to induce labor or abortion, but is often used in anesthesia to help the uterine contract to decrease bleeding postpartum. It is a prostaglandin (PGE1) that can also help to keep a PDA open until surgical correction.

Antiarrhythmic Drug Classes

Sodium Channel Blockers (Class Ia - Ic)
Beta-Adrenergic Blockers (Class II)
Potassium Channel Blockers (Class III)
Calcium Channel Blockers (Class IV)

Class Ia

Double **Q**uarter **P**ounder
Disopyramide
Quinidine
Procainamide

Class Ib

With **L**ettuce, **M**ayo, and **T**omato
Lidocaine
Mexeletine
Tocainide

Class Ic

And **M**ore **F**ries **P**lease
Moricizine
Flecainide
Propefanone

Class II

<u>LOL</u>
Proprano**lol**
Ateno**lol**
Metopro**lol**

Class III

<u>SAD</u>
Sotalol
Amiodarone
Dofelitide

Class IV

Venereal **Di**sease
Verapamil
Diltiazem

Medication Dosing by Weight

[Meds Dosed by Total Body Weight]

Specific **P**ounds

Succinylcholine, **P**ropofol (TIVA)

[Meds Dosed by Lean Body Weight]

Fewer **R**eal **P**ounds

Fentanyl, **R**emifentanil, **P**ropofol (Induction)

[Meds Does by Ideal Body Weight]

CARVE the fat

Cisatracurium

Atracurium

Rocuronium

Vecuronium

Neuromuscular Blockers That Cause Histamine Release

hi**STAM**ine

Sux

Tubocurarine

Atracurium

Mivacurium

Histamine release can create a problem, as it often causes hypotension, tachycardia, flushing, and bronchospasm in asthmatics. Tubocurarine is no longer used, and you are unlikely to see Mivacurium either. However, it is common to have test questions with these drugs on them.

Anesthesia
Basics

Guedel's Stages of Anesthesia

Induce Every One Delicately

Stage 1: Induction

Stage 2: Excitement

Stage 3: Operative

Stage 4: Danger

The first stage occurs from the beginning of the induction of anesthesia to the loss of consciousness. Patient's may still feel pain, as this is the lightest stage. Stage 2 requires great vigilance, as this is the point at which several things may happen. Blood pressure and heart rate increase and stimulation may cause muscle irritation, specifically with the airway. Watch out for laryngospasm in this stage! Stage 3 is where we want to be while operating. The patient is not too deep or too light, but there is little or no response to surgical stimulation. Stage 4 means that you have gone too far. You may see a decrease in blood pressure, as well as respirations if the patient isn't being mechanically ventilated. If not treated or reversed quickly, this can eventually lead to death.

Factors that don't affect MAC

LIGHT

Length of anesthesia
Inhaled gas metabolism
Gender
Hyperkalemia/Hypokalemia
Thyroid Dysfunction

The MAC (minimum alveolar concentration) of inhaled anesthetics will not be increased or decreased by these factors. The amount of time that a patient is under anesthesia is irrelevant, as is the rate of metabolism of any gas. When all else is equal, a female will require just as much or as little anesthesia as a male. Potassium and thyroid dysfunction also do not affect MAC requirements.

Factors that increase MAC

CHILD

Chronic ethanol abuse

Hyperthermia, **H**ypernatremia

Infants 6-12 months

Locks of Red (Red Hair)

Drugs that increase catecholamine levels

Chronic alcoholics have typically been able to build up a tolerance to the depressant effects of the alcohol, and therefore anesthetics. Patients with a high temperature, increased sodium level, and those with red hair may require an increased MAC (minimum alveolar concentration). MAC requirement peaks at the age of 6-12 months, and then gradually decreases as we get older. Patients who are getting drugs that increase catecholamine levels may also require more gas. Examples of this include MAO inhibitors, cocaine, ephedrine, and levodopa.

Factors that decrease MAC

HAPPINESS

Hypothermia
Alpha agonists
Pre-op meds
Pregnancy
Induced hypotension
Neonates
Elderly
Sodium low
Stoned

Many factors can decrease the MAC (minimum alveolar concentration) requirements, including hypothermia. You may see a 2-5% decrease per Celsius degree drop. Alpha agonists, such as clonidine and Precedex, may also cause a decrease. Pre-operative medications, such as fentanyl and versed, pregnancy, induced hypotension, and hyponatremia are all something to consider. Neonates have a decreased MAC requirement until around 6 months of age. It will then increase for a few months before beginning its decline as they get older. About a 6% decrease in MAC requirements can be expected per decade of life, which is why the elderly don't require as much anesthesia. Patients who have taken drugs or alcohol shortly before surgery will likely require less anesthesia as well.

Receptor blockade

100%: flaccid; no responses; no TOF
95%: No twitches but diaphragm may move
90%: 1 twitch on TOF; adequate relaxation for abd. Procedures
70%: 4 twitches on TOF; VC and TV can be normal
50%: can pass inspiratory pressure test
30%: Head lift/hand grasp sustained

A silly rhyme to help you remember:

-At one hundred percent, no response is sent
-At ninety-five, only the diaphragm is live
-Down five more, there's 1 on the train-of-four
-At a block of seven zero, you're a 4 twitch hero
-At a 50 percent block, the inspiratory pressure test is a lock
-Once you get to thirty, their head will be sturdy

Muscarinic Effects of Acetylcholine

She **L**ooks **DUMB**

Salivation

Lacrimation

Defecation

Urination

Miosis

Bradycardia, **B**ronchoconstriction

Anticholinesterase drugs, such as Neostigmine, are responsible for preventing the breakdown of acetylcholine, thereby making more of it available. Because of this, giving such a medication will yield results such as those listed above. This is why it is important to also use an anticholinergic, such as glycopyrrolate, to help counteract these effects.

Plasma Membrane Function

PACTS

Protection

Activation of receptors

Cell-to-cell communication

Transportation

Structure

If your anesthesia program requires a chemistry or biology component, then you are likely to see a question regarding the plasma membrane. There is nothing in-depth here—just a basic overview of its functions.

Fluid Maintenance During Surgery

You must take into account the hourly maintenance fluids, plus fluids that the patient will need due to being NPO, as well as those to replace fluid shifts during surgery.

Hourly Maintenance

4-2-1 Rule

4 cc/kg/hr first 10 kg of body weight
2 cc/kg/hr second 10 kg of body weight
1 cc/kg/hr for the remaining weight in kg

For example, here's the calculation for a 75 kg patient:
4 x 10 = 40
2 x 10 = 20
1 x 55 = 55
Total = 115 cc/hr

Shortcut: (Pt's weight in kg) + 40

NPO Deficit

(Number of hours NPO) x (Hourly maintenance rate)

50% during the first hour
25% in the 2nd hour
25% in the 3rd hour

For example, here is the calculation for our 75 kg patient who has been NPO for 12 hours:

12 x 115 (from calc. above) = 1380 mL

690 mL in the 1st hour
345 mL in the 2nd hour
345 mL in the 3rd hour

Intra-operative Fluid Shifts

Small Incision/minimal trauma: 2-4 cc/kg/hr
Moderate Incision/moderate trauma: 4-6 cc/kg/hr
Large/Incision/severe trauma: 6-8 cc/kg/hr
Major vascular case/extreme trauma: 8-10 cc/kg/hr

Allowable Blood Loss

This is a good calculation to help you decide when you should consider transfusion of blood products.

Maximum Allowable Blood Loss (MABL)

[(Existing Hct – Desired Hct)/Existing Hct] X [Body wt/kg x EBV]

For example:
[(45g/dl-30g/dl) / 45 g/dl] x [70 kg x 75 kg/mL]
= [(15 g/dL) / 45 g/dL] x [5250mL]
= 0.33 x 5250 mL
= 1750 ml

*Estimated Blood Volume (EBV)
Premature Neonates: 95 ml/kg
Term Neonates: 85 ml/kg
Infants & Children: 80 ml/kg
Adult Males: 75 ml/kg
Adult Females: 65 ml/kg

Vertebrae

33 vertebrae

7 Cervical
12 Thoracic
5 Lumbar
5 Sacral
4 Coccygeal

Mnemonic:

Breakfast at **7** (Cervical)
Lunch at **12** (Thoracic)
Dinner at **5** (Lumbar)

5 people eating at a **4**-person table makes for a tight fit (Sacral and Coccygeal)

"Tight fit" because they are fused together.
Coccyx is commonly 4, but can be between 3-5

Pharmacokinetics

ADME

Absorption
Distribution
Metabolism
Excretion

Absorption: When a drug enters the bloodstream
Distribution: The movement of a drug throughout the body once in the bloodstream
Metabolism: The body uses the drug and gives off a byproduct
Excretion: Getting rid of the byproduct from the body

Drug Interactions: Additive, Synergistic, Antagonistic

Additive: **Add**

Additive: Adding 2 or more substances together to get a total effect that is equal to sum of the individual effects (1+1 = 2).

Sy**nerg**istic: Synergy = more e**nerg**y

Synergistic: Interaction between 2 or more substances to get a total effect that is greater than the sum of the individual effects (1+1 = 3).

Antagonistic: **Anti**

Antagonistic: Interaction between 2 or more substances in which the effect of either is diminished (1+1 = 0).

Gas Laws

<u>C</u>an <u>T</u>hese <u>G</u>uys <u>P</u>ossibly <u>B</u>e <u>V</u>iolinists

<u>C</u>harles

<u>T</u>emperature

<u>G</u>ay-Lussac

<u>P</u>ressure

<u>B</u>oyle

<u>V</u>olume

Charles' Law: When pressure is constant, volume and temperature are *directly* proportional.

Gay-Lussac's Law: When volume is constant, pressure and temperature are *directly* proportional.

Boyles' Law: When temperature is constant, pressure and volume are *inversely* proportional.

Inhalationals – MAC Value

-Listed from Lowest to Highest

I **S**carf **D**esserts **N**ightly

Isoflurane

Sevoflurane

Desflurane

Nitrous Oxide

A low MAC value simply means that the gas is more potent and less is needed. Isoflurane has a MAC value around 1.2, Sevoflurane around 2.0, and Desflurane around 6.6. Nitrous Oxide has a MAC value around 104%, meaning that you can never have enough to get to 1 MAC.

Dermatomes

C4: C for **C**ollar

T4: **T**eats (nipples)

L4: Four-letter word for the **L**eg (Knee)

S4: **S**it on it (Butt)

This should help guide you to give you at least a rough idea of what the rest of the dermatomes represent. I would still recommend trying to memorize the dermatome map to the best of your ability. But you can always go back to one of these to bring you to the right area of the body.

Fire Triad

Hall **O**f **F**ame

Heat (Ignition source)

Oxidizer

Fuel

For a fire to happen, all three of these things must be present. Examples of ignition sources are lasers, drills, and electrocautery units. An oxidizer could be oxygen or nitrous oxide. Examples of Fuels include tracheal tubes, sponges, and drapes.

Pre-anesthetic Assessment

A - Affirmative history: Details of past illness and treatment.
A - Airway: Detailed airway examination.

B - Blood hemoglobin, blood loss estimation, and blood availability: Check for hemoglobin level, calculate the maximum allowable blood loss, and make sure blood is available if needed.
B - Breathing: Check respiratory rate and breathing pattern.

C - Clinical examination: Assess pulse, rhythm, blood pressure, and oxygen saturation.
C - Co-morbidities: Check for diseases such as diabetes, hypertension, asthma, and epilepsy.

D – Drugs: Find out which medications are being taken by the patient and determine how they may or may not affect your anesthesia plan.
D - Details of previous anesthesia and surgeries: Make sure patients haven't had any problems with anesthesia in the past and check to see what kinds of surgeries they have had.

E - Evaluate Studies: Look for appropriate studies that have been done that may help guide anesthetic management.
E - End point to take up the case for surgery: There should be an end point to take up the case for surgery to avoid unnecessary postponement if further optimization is not possible.

F - Fluid status: Determine how long it's been since the patient had any fluids and look for signs of dehydration.
F - Fasting: Make sure the patient has been fasting an appropriate amount of time.

G - Give physical status: Assign a physical status classification.
G - Get consent: Discuss the anesthetic risk with the patient to obtain appropriate consent.

Pain

Nociception – Processes

Totally Treat My Pain

Transduction
Transmission
Modulation
Perception

Nociception is basically the ability to feel pain, which is caused by stimulation of a nociceptor. It is comprised of four main processes: transduction, transmission, modulation, and perception. Transduction is the conversion of stimuli by a nociceptor into electrical energy. Transmission is the movement of the stimulus through the peripheral nervous system using first order neurons. Modulation is the transfer of the stimulus from the first order neurons to the second order neurons in the spinal cord. Perception is how the signal is perceived by the brain. In order to prevent or treat pain, one of these processes must be disrupted.

Opioid receptors

Mu-1: **MUSE**

Miosis
Urinary retention
Supraspinal analgesia (mostly)
Euphoria

Mu-2: **BRAINS**

Bradycardia
Respiratory depression
Addiction
Itching
Nausea/vomiting/constipation
Spinal analgesia (mostly)

Kappa (κ): **S**ame **S**hit, **D**ifferent **D**ay

Spinal analgesia (mostly)
Sedation
Dysphoria
Dependence

Delta (δ): **RAPS**

Respiratory depression
Addiction
Poorly understood

Supraspinal/Spinal analgesia

Double check this against the educational material from your institution. There are different functions cited on a few different sources. Study the material you have been given and tweak the mnemonics accordingly.

Opioids (from most to least potent)

Superman **R**escued **F**ive **A**merican **H**orses
Monday **M**orning

Sufentanil > **R**emifentanil = **F**entanyl > **A**lfentanil
> **H**ydromorphone > **M**orphine > **M**eperidine

Sufentanil is almost 10 times more potent than
Fentanyl, while Remifentanil's potency matches
closely with Fentanyl's. Fentanyl is 5-10 times more
potent than Alfentanil. Hydromorphone is 8-10 times
more potent than Morphine, but Morphine is 10
times more potent than Meperidine.

Central opioid effects vs peripheral opioid effects

Central Opioid Effects

MARS

Miosis, **M**ood alteration
Analgesia
Respiratory depression
Sedation

Peripheral Opioid Effects

SHIV

Smooth muscle contraction
Histamine release
Inhibition of acetylcholine release
Venous dilatation

Complications

Pulmonary Embolism (PE) – Treatment

FATS

Filter (IVC filter)

Anticoagulants

Thrombolytics

Symptoms (Treat symptoms – oxygen, pain meds, CPR, vent)

Pulmonary embolisms happen suddenly and can lead to death very quickly. Even with fast treatment, it's often not enough to stop these. Once a PE happens, all you can do is treat the symptoms and begin life-saving measures until the patient is stabilized. If a patient has a known history of DVT or PE, then other preventative options can be put in place, such as an IVC filter, anticoagulants, and thrombolytics.

Malignant Hyperthermia - Symptoms

MATH

Muscle Spasms
Acidosis (Rapid increase in EtCO2)
Tachycardia
Hyperthermia

Alternative...

IM STAT

Increased EtCO2, Temperature

Muscle rigidity

Sweating

Tachycardia

Acidosis (metabolic and respiratory)

Tachypnea

Often, the first clinical sign you'll see is a rapid increase in end-tidal CO2. Once you see this, start thinking about malignant hyperthermia. You will also see the tachycardia, tachypnea, and muscle rigidity. The other symptoms will follow quickly, so treatment must begin as soon as it's recognized. All inhalational anesthetics are known triggers for MH, as well as succinylcholine. Anyone who has a personal or family history of MH should have these things nowhere near the operating room. A new machine and circuit without attached gases should be used in these patients.

Malignant Hyperthermia - Treatment

Cool SODA

Cool the patient (ice lavage, ice packs, etc.)

Sodium Bicarb
Oxygen (Hyperventilate)
Dantrolene
Agents Off

As soon as malignant hyperthermia is recognized, treatment must be started right away. The first thing you do is notify the surgeon and call for help. While you are waiting, turn the agents off and switch to 100% oxygen. There should be a malignant hyperthermia cart with everything you need in it. When help arrives, start mixing and administering the Dantrolene. Have the OR staff cool the patient however possible, including ice water in the surgical site and ice packs all around the patient's body. You can use ice water to lavage the stomach through an OG tube. Keep the treatments going for as long as it takes until the patient is stable or is no longer viable.

Cholinergic syndrome (Cholinergic Crisis) - Symptoms

Beach CLAMS

Bronchoconstriction, Bradycardia

Confusion, Coma
Lethargy
Abdominal cramping
Miosis
Salivation, Seizure

Or...

SLUDGE

Salivation
Lacrimation (tearing)
Urination
Diarrhea
GI Distress
Emesis

These symptoms are an extreme form of those that happen with anticholinesterase drugs, such as Neostigmine. Although the dosing of the reversal agents we give are usually too small, it is possible, and you should be able to recognize it when you see it. A common cause of this syndrome is organophosphate poisoning.

Cholinergic syndrome (Cholinergic Crisis) - Treatment

IPAD

Intubation (if respiratory arrest occurs)

Pralidoxime

Atropine

Diazepam (benzos)

Treatment for cholinergjc crisis starts with Atropine, an anticholinergic, and Pralidoxime, an oxime that helps bind to the acetylcholinesterase that has been inactivated by organophosphate. Edrophonium has also been used. Diazepam is helpful when used in conjunction with Atropine. Respiratory insufficiency or complete arrest is common due to paralysis of the respiratory muscles. Intubation may be necessary while stabilizing the patient.

Anticholinergic syndrome - Symptoms

DARTH VADER

Dry Mouth, **D**ry flushed skin
Agitation
Rash (Face, neck, chest)
Tachycardia
Hallucinations, **H**yperthermia

Vision blurred
Asleep (Drowsy)
Disoriented
Excitement (Mania)
Reduced Blood pressure (Hypotension)

Alternative...

Hot as a Hare (Hyperthermia)
Mad as a Hatter (Confusion, delirium)
Red as a Beet (Flushed face, rash)
Dry as a Bone (decreased secretions, thirsty)
Blind as a Bat (Blurred vision)

*Treatment for anticholinergic syndrome is Physostigmine

Venous Air Embolism (VAE) - Symptoms

SHAME

Sats Decreased

Hypotension

Arrhythmia

Millwheel Murmur

EtCO2 sudden drop

Similar to a pulmonary embolism, a venous air embolism happens suddenly and without warning. There will usually be a sudden decrease in end-tidal CO2, along with extreme hypotension. Soon after, the oxygen saturation will drop and you may see arrhythmias. Death is often the end result when not recognized and treated quickly. Although you may not have time to listen for it, you can often hear a millwheel murmur, which can help diagnose VAE if you aren't sure.

Venous Air Embolism - Treatment

BAD HOP

Bone wax
Aspirate through CVP
Durant's Maneuver

Hydrate (give fluids)
Oxygen
Pressors

Alternative...

GAS OD

Give Pressors
Aspirate via right heart catheter (if available)
Stop Nitrous Oxide

Oxygen (100%)
Durant's Maneuver

Durant's Maneuver is putting the patient into a Trendelenburg and left lateral position. Doing this might help to get the entrained air bubble to move inside the right ventricle, no longer causing an obstruction. The withdrawal of venous air can be performed if the patient has a central venous catheter. If it progresses to cardiac arrest, direct needle puncture of the right heart has been advocated by some to sustain circulation.

Local Anesthetic Toxicity

CLUSTER FUC*

Circumoral (and tongue) numbness
Lightheadedness
Unconsciousness
Seizures
Tinnitus, twitching (muscles)
Eyesight disturbances
Respiratory arrest

Fibrillation (arrhythmias)
Urticaria
Cardiovascular collapse
***

Or...

MASS

Muscle twitching
Altered Central Nervous System (dizzy, drowsy, confused)
Slurred or difficult speech (circumoral and tongue numbness)
Seizures

Monitoring and Equipment

CVP Tracing

A Wave: **A**trial (Right atrial contraction)
C Wave: **C**ontraction (Isovolumic ventricular contraction)
V Wave: **V**enous (Venous return against closed tricuspid valve)

The CVP parallels right atrial pressure, something that is influenced by the volume in the right ventricle. A normal CVP waveform consists of three peaks (a,c,v waves) and two descents (x,y). The A wave represents right atrial contraction and occurs just after the P wave on the ECG. It is absent in a-fib and may be exaggerated with junctional rhythms. The C wave represents isovolumic ventricular contraction, which forces the tricuspid valve to bulge upward into the right atrium. The V wave represents venous return against the closed tricuspid valve. You will likely see large V waves with tricuspid regurgitation.

EEG Waveforms

Alpha: **ACE** (**A**wake, **C**losed **E**yes)

Beta: **Be T**otally **A**wake (normal awake)

Delta: **D**eep sleep

Theta: **The T**ypical **A**sleep state

The alpha waveform on an EEG is seen when the patient is awake, but with their eyes closed. The beta waveform is seen when the patient is awake with their eyes open. The delta wave will be seen after the patient enters a deep sleep state. The theta waveform is present when the patient is in a normal sleep state (not too deep and not too light).

Neuromonitoring: Effects from Anesthesia

(From most sensitive to least sensitive)

My **V**olatiles **S**hock **B**rains

MEPs (Motor Evoked Potentials)

VEPs (Visual Evoked Potentials)

SSEPs (Somatosensory Evoked Potentials)

BAEPs (Brainstem Auditory Evoked Potentials)

Motor Evoked Potentials (MEPs) are the *most* sensitive to the effects of anesthesia, while Brainstem Auditory Evoked Potentials (BAEPs) are the *least* sensitive.

Mapleson systems – Order of Efficiency

(Most efficient to least efficient)

-Spontaneous Ventilation

All **D**ogs **C**an **B**ite

A > **D** > **C/B**

-Controlled Ventilation

Dead **B**odies **C**an't **A**rgue

D > **B/C** > **A**

Equipment Set-Up

SOAP ME

Suction
Oxygen
Airway
Pharmaceuticals

Monitors
Equipment

Check the wall suction and back-up cylinders and make sure there is an ambu/mask in room. Attach and check the circuit, calibrate the O2 analyzer, and test the flow meters. Perform a leak test, check the scavenger system and ventilator. Get your oral airways, laryngoscope, blades, and ET tube with stylet and syringe. Check your blades and ETT balloon. If needed, have things ready like an OG tube and esophageal stethoscope.

Make sure the EKG, pulse ox, and blood pressure cuff are ready to go and easily accessible. A twitch monitor should be available, gel pads for the EKG, and anything else you may need. Consider what other equipment might be necessary, such as transducers/cables for a-line/CVP/swan, fluid/blood warmer, spinal/epidural kit, Bair hugger, chest rolls, prone pillow, blankets, head rest for positioning, pumps, external pacer/defibrillator, or BIS monitor.

Equipment Check Prior to Induction

MALES

Mask/Ambu

Airways

Laryngoscopes

Endotracheal tubes

Suction/**S**tylette

Before at induction, you should have these basic supplies ready in your room. It doesn't matter if you are only doing light sedation or general anesthesia. You must always be ready for general anesthesia in case things go sideways. Have your suction ready and easily accessible, and an ambu available just in case. Have an endotracheal tube ready with a stylette in place. Make sure the blade is attached to the laryngoscopes handle and the light is functional. You should also have oral airways available in case you have difficulty ventilating.

Regional
Anesthesia

Epidurals – Structures the Needle Will Pass Through

From posterior to anterior:

The **Sk**eleton **Sub**dues **Sup**erman's **I**tchy **L**eg **E**very **S**aturday

Skin
SubQ tissue
Supraspinous ligament
Intraspinous ligament
Ligamentum flavum
Epidural space
Spinal meninges

Layers of the spinal meninges:

Dutch **A**pple **P**ie

Dura mater
Arachnoid mater
Pia mater

Spinal Contraindications

CHAIR

Coagulopathies

Hypovolemic shock

Aortic Stenosis (severe)

Increased ICP/Infection at site of injection

Refusal by patient

Many people consider patient refusal the only absolute contraindication to spinal anesthesia. However, all of these things should be taken into account when considering whether or not to do the procedure. Weigh the benefits versus the risks before proceeding.

Order of Spinal Blockade

Soft **T**oilet **P**aper **T**ouches **P**eru's **M**ost **V**aluable
People

S-T-P-T-P-M-V-P
Sympathetic
Temperature
Pain
Touch
Pressure
Motor
Vibration
Proprioception

The first thing to be affected by spinal anesthesia
is the sympathetic nervous system, followed by
sensation to temperature and pain perception.
Soon after, patients are unable to sense that you
are touching them or applying pressure.
Eventually, they won't be able to move the
affected area, and they will lose the sense of
vibration and proprioception.

Anatomical Structures – Order of Vascularity

More vascular to less vascular order. The more vascular something is, the greater the risk of toxicity from local anesthetics.

BICEPSS

Blood/Tracheal
Intercostal
Caudal/Paracervical
Epidural
Plexus (Brachial)
Spinal
Subcutaneous

Spinal Needle Characteristics

Quincke: **Cut**ting

Sprotte, **W**hitacre: **Pencil**-point

Quitters like to take short-**Cut**s

School **W**ork needs a **Pencil**

The incidence of Post-Dural Puncture Headache
(PDPH) is higher with the use of a cutting needle,
such as the Quincke. A pencil point needle will
separate the fibers, rather than cut them,
thereby reducing this risk.

Local Anesthetics – Hyperbaric vs Isobaric vs Hypobaric

Hyperbaric: Density > CSF
Hyper: **More** Dense

Hypobaric: Density < CSF
Hypo: **Less** Dense

Isobaric: Density = CSF
Iso: **Same** Density

A hyperbaric local anesthetic will have more density than CSF. Therefore, it will sink to the bottom and follow gravity. Hypobaric solutions are less dense than CSF, so they will rise. Isobaric solutions have the same density as CSF, so will generally stay where injected.

Places to Avoid Epinephrine with Local Anesthetic

Nose

Hose

Fingers

and

Toes

Infiltration of local anesthesia with epinephrine increases the risk for local ischemic necrosis in distal structures such as these. Hose = Penis, in case you haven't figured it out by now.

Local Anesthetic Protein Binding (Short to Long)

Pretty Cheerleaders Like My Round Butt Every Time

Procaine

Chloroprocaine

Lidocaine

Mepivacaine

Ropivacaine

Bupivacaine

Etidocaine

Tetracaine

MORE

CRNA

MNEMONICS

125 MORE TIPS, TRICKS, AND MEMORY CUES TO HELP YOU KICK-ASS IN CRNA SCHOOL

Chris Mulder, CRNA, MSN

Airway

Hypocapnia - Causes

Hyper CHAD

Hyperventilation

Cold

Hypotension

Anesthesia

Dead space ventilation decreased

Hypocapnia is when the CO_2 levels in the body fall to below normal levels and can be caused by many factors. Hyperventilation is a common culprit, whether this be by means of voluntary or mechanical ventilation. It can also be the result of decreased CO_2 production (hypothermia, deep anesthesia, hypotension) and decreased dead space ventilation (decreased PEEP, decreased rebreathing, etc). It may be seen in hypothermia or during periods of hypotension. By far the most common cause of hypocapnia is hyperventilation by mechanical means.

Hypercapnia - Causes

CHI

CO2 absorber exhausted

Hypoventilation

Increased dead space ventilation

Hypercapnia is the increase of carbon dioxide in the body above normal levels. Anything that produces more CO2 can be the cause of hypercapnia. For example, you might see it when the CO2 absorber is exhausted, during hypoventilation (depression of ventilation by drugs such as opioids), or when there is an increase in dead space ventilation.

Post-intubation Croup – Risk Factors

HELPER

Head and neck procedures

Early childhood (14 years or less)

Large endotracheal tube

Prolonged surgery

Excessive movement of the endotracheal tube

Repeated intubation attempts

Croup in the post-surgical patient who was intubated is caused by tracheal or glottic edema. There are many things that may play a role, increasing the risk. For example, any procedure that is done in the head and neck area could be the culprit. A large endotracheal tube, excessive movement of the tube, or repeated intubation attempts will all cause irritation to the trachea and glottic opening. Prolonged surgery may also increase the risk for post-intubation croup, as does being a child. Sometimes, it is just going to happen regardless of any precautions, but try to be aware of the common risk factors and adjust appropriately.

One-Lung Ventilation – Absolute Indications

Confine **S**ingle **L**ung **F**irst

Cysts or unilateral bullae

Secretions in one lung

Lavage

Fistula

Although one-lung ventilation is usually voluntary to facilitate surgery, it is sometimes necessary due to other factors. For example, if a patient has cysts or bullae on one side, they may rupture during positive pressure ventilation. Also, contamination of both lungs could be deadly, so blood or infectious secretions in one lung indicates the need for lung isolation. If bronchopulmonary lavage is being done, it is needed to prevent spilling over of fluid to the nondependent lung. Lastly, a bronchopleural fistula or a bronchocutaneous fistula mandates one-lung ventilation.

Increase in Dead Space

APPLE

Age

Positive-pressure ventilation

Pulmonary embolism

Lung disease

Extension of Neck/Jaw

Dead space is the portion of air that is inhaled (or delivered), but doesn't participate in gas exchange. This could be caused by many things, and is increased by age, positive-pressure ventilation, pulmonary embolism, lung disease, and extension of the neck and jaw. Another common thing that increases dead space is the breathing circuit. The longer the circuit, the more dead space there is. This air basically gets wasted, doing neither harm nor good.

Trans-tracheal Jet Ventilation – Complications

SAME BED

Subcutaneous emphysema
Arterial perforation
Mediastinal emphysema
Exhalation difficulty

Barotrauma
Esophageal puncture
Damage to tracheal mucosa

Trans-tracheal jet ventilation is sometimes used when difficult airways are expected or in certain surgical procedures when very low tidal volumes are needed. It is not very common, but it's important to know the potential complications when you are faced with this challenge. Barotrauma can result in pneumothorax, while air can also enter as subcutaneous emphysema or mediastinal emphysema. Arterial perforation and damage to the tracheal mucosa is a potential complication, as is esophageal puncture, which will result in bleeding and hemoptysis.

Fiberoptic Bronchoscopy - Contraindications

BLUSH

Bleeding

Local Anesthetic Allergy

Unable to Cooperate

Secretions

Hypoxia

While fiberoptic bronchoscopy may be useful in many situations, it is also contraindicated under certain circumstances. If a patient is bleeding from any part of the airway and is not resolved with suction, you might want to put the scope down. Hypoxia and heavy airway secretions (even after suction and antisialagogues) are also a contraindication. For an awake fiberoptic attempt, the patient should be able to cooperate and receive local anesthesia. If not, you should probably consider another way.

Pulse Oximetry Artifact – Low Perfusion States

HAIL

Hypothermia

Anemia

Increased systemic vascular resistance

Low cardiac output

Pulse oximetry artifact can be caused by a few different things, including electrical interference, moving/shaking, malfunction, and low perfusion states. Hypothermia, anemia, increased systemic vascular resistance, and low cardiac output are all examples of low perfusion states that may cause pulse oximetry artifact. One way to get a better reading on the monitor is to place the probe in a better perfused area, such as the earlobe or forehead.

PEEP – Potential Disadvantages

RIP

Redistribution of pulmonary blood flow

Increased extravascular lung water

Pulmonary barotrauma

PEEP is positive end-expiratory pressure, something that can be very beneficial for certain patient populations and in certain situations. But it can have potential disadvantages also. PEEP can cause redistribution of pulmonary blood flow from the core to the periphery. It may also cause increased extravascular lung water, which is the fluid that accumulates in the alveolar and interstitial spaces. Another issue could be pulmonary barotrauma if the PEEP and tidal volume are too much for the patient's lungs.

Gas Flow Obstruction – Typical Causes

<u>B</u>ECK

Blood or secretions in the ETT

Expiratory valve malfunction

Cuff herniation

Kinking of the ETT

There aren't many things more annoying than hearing a high-pressure alarm from the ventilator, and can be quite nerve racking when you can't figure out the source of the problem. There may be several reasons for gas flow obstruction, but some common ones include kinking of the ET tube, blood/secretions in the ET tube, expiratory valve malfunction, and cuff herniation. Cuff herniation is possible if it is overinflated (if it doesn't rupture), going over the ET tube, effectively blocking it. You would also get the high-pressure alarm if the patient is coughing or pushing against the vent, having a bronchospasm, or if a mucous plug is present.

Cardiovascular System

Histamine - Cardiovascular Effects

CRIES

Chronotropic

Relaxes smooth muscles

Inotropic

Edema

Stimulates adrenal medulla

Histamine has many effects in the body, and the cardiovascular system is no different. When it's released, either from natural reasons or from medications, the heart rate increases (chronotropic) and the smooth muscles of arterioles and small blood vessels relax (hypotension). It also causes edema by increasing capillary permeability, as well as stimulating the adrenal medulla to release catecholamines.

Fat Embolism Syndrome – Symptom Triad

Come Help Please

Confusion

Hypoxemia

Petechiae

Fat embolism syndrome is a potential complication with fractures or during orthopedic surgery. Three of the most common symptoms are hypoxemia, petechia, and confusion or respiratory distress (in awake patients). If these three symptoms present, along with orthopedic involvement, then it would be wise to suspect fat embolism syndrome.

Idiopathic Subaortic Stenosis – Drugs to Avoid

Don't **P**oke **B**oob **V**eins

Diuretics

Positive inotropes

Beta adrenergic agonists

Vasodilators

Idiopathic subaortic stenosis is a type of left ventricular outflow obstruction. Certain medications should be avoided in patients with this condition, as they can sometimes worsen the obstruction. These agents include diuretics, beta adrenergic agonists, positive inotropes (calcium, digitalis), and vasodilators (nitroprusside, nitroglycerine). Sorry for the randomness of this mnemonic, but I'll bet you won't forget Don't Poke Boob Veins.

Vasospasm – H Therapy

Hypervolemia

Hemodilution

Hypertension

When a patient is having a vasospasm, 'H' therapy can be a successful treatment. Colloids and Crystalloids should be given aggressively to keep the CVP higher than 10 mmHg or the PCWP 12-20 mmHg. Be careful not to put the patient into congestive heart failure. They should also be hemodiluted to a hematocrit of around 33 percent. This can help to balance viscosity and oxygen-carrying capacity. Hypertension should also be a goal by using agents such as dopamine, phenylephrine, and dobutamine. The systolic blood pressure should be maintained around 160-200 mmHg.

Hypotension During Surgery - Causes

<u>CVS D</u>rugs

<u>C</u>ontractility (Decreased)

<u>V</u>enous return (Preload – Decreased)

<u>S</u>ystemic vascular resistance (Decreased)

<u>D</u>ysrhythmias

Hypotension is a common occurrence while a patient is under anesthesia. While we know that a bleeding patient or dehydrated patient will drop their blood pressure, you should know the basic physiologic reasons. Common causes include decreased contractility, decreased systemic vascular resistance, and dysrhythmias. A decreased preload will also cause hypotension.

Air Embolism – Treatment

DARES

Durant Maneuver

Aspiration

Release Pneumoperitoneum

Eliminate Nitrous Oxide

Stop Insufflation

Air embolism during surgery is a very dangerous thing that must be acted upon quickly. Make the surgeon aware of the situation, have them stop the insufflation, and release the peritoneum. If you have nitrous oxide running, turn it off. If the patient has a central line, you can try aspirating the air from the right atrium. You can also try repositioning, using the Durant Maneuver, putting the patient in a left-lateral tilt and Trendelenburg.

Air Embolism – Detection (Intermediate Sensitivity)

Put some **PEP** in your step

Pulmonary artery pressure

End-tidal CO2

PaO2

Early treatment of air embolism is extremely important. But before treatment can be started, the problem must first be identified. The patient will have a decreased PaO2, decreased end-tidal CO2, and an elevated pulmonary artery pressure. These forms of detection are considered to be intermediate sensitivity.

Pulmonary Embolism – Treatment

O SHIT

Oxygen

Support cardiovascular function

Heparin

Intubate if necessary

Treat hypotension

If you're ever faced with the terrifying situation of an intraoperative pulmonary embolism, it is important to know how to respond quickly. The first thing is to treat the symptoms that are presenting in the moment and if it's a big PE, making sure they don't die. You might just be in ACLS mode at this point. In general, though, you will want to give more oxygen and intubate if necessary, treat hypotension and support cardiovascular function, and start the patient on anticoagulation once stable.

Hepatic Artery and Portal Vein – Receptors

Hepatic Artery:

ABCD

Alpha-1 (vasoconstriction)
Beta-2 (vasodilation)
Cholinergic (vasodilation)
D1 (vasodilation)

Portal Vein:

AD

Alpha-1 (vasoconstriction)
D1 (vasodilation)

In the liver, the hepatic artery and portal vein have receptors that each function to cause either vasodilation or vasoconstriction, among other things. Alpha-1 and D1 receptors can be found on both the hepatic artery and portal vein. Alpha-1 causes vasoconstriction, while D1 causes vasodilation. Beta-2 receptors and cholinergic receptors are found on the hepatic artery and they both cause vasodilation.

Myocardial Oxygen Demand – Determining Factors

CHAP

Contractility

Heart rate

Afterload

Preload

Myocardial oxygen demand is increased when more of it is being used. The factors that determine this include contractility, heart rate, afterload, and preload. Afterload is the systolic wall tension, while preload is the diastolic wall tension. When one of these factors is increased, the myocardial oxygen consumption is also increased, thereby increasing myocardial oxygen demand. On the other hand, when one of these factors is decreased, oxygen consumption is also decreased, thereby decreasing myocardial oxygen demand.

Myocardial Oxygen Supply – Determining Factors

HALO

Heart Rate

Aortic Diastolic Pressure

Left Ventricular End-diastolic Pressure

Oxygen Content/**O**xygen Extraction

Myocardial oxygen supply is determined by several factors. A high heart rate could lower perfusion because of the decrease in the diastole time (when coronary blood flow occurs). If the aortic diastolic pressure is low, then perfusion pressure is low. A high left ventricular end-diastolic pressure could decrease flow by compressing the subendocardium. Lastly, myocardial oxygen supply is determined by the obvious: the amount of oxygen content in arterial blood and the amount of oxygen being extracted.

Aortic Stenosis – Hemodynamic Goals

Silly Full Time RN

Slow (low heart rate)

Full (maintained or increased preload)

Tight (maintained or increased afterload - SVR)

Regular (maintain sinus rhythm)

Not too strong (maintain contractility).

A major goal with aortic stenosis patients is to not let the heart rate increase. You'll also want to maintain or even increase the preload (Full), maintain or increase the afterload (Tight), keep them in normal sinus rhythm (Regular), and maintain the contractility (Not too strong). AS: Always Slow.

Aortic Insufficiency – Hemodynamic Goals

Fat, Fake, Farting **RN**

Fast (high heart rate)

Full (increase preload)

Forward (decrease afterload)

Regular (maintain sinus rhythm)

Not too strong (maintain contractility)

When you are encountered with a patient who has aortic insufficiency, remember first and foremost to keep the heart rate up (Fast). You should also make it a goal to increase the preload (Full), decrease the afterload (Forward), keep them in normal sinus rhythm (Regular), and maintain the contractility (Not too strong). AI: Always Increased.

Valvular Heart Disease – Cardiac Parameters to Monitor

PARCH

Preload

Afterload (determined by SVR)

Rhythm

Contractility

Heart rate

While taking care of a patient who has existing valvular heart disease, there are several cardiac parameters that should be monitored, especially while under anesthesia. These monitors include preload, afterload, rhythm, contractility, and heart rate.

Mitral Stenosis – Hemodynamic Goals

Silly Night Nurse RN

Slow (low heart rate)

Not too full (maintained preload)

Not too tight (maintained afterload (SVR)

Regular (maintain sinus rhythm)

Not too strong (maintained contractility)

Patients with mitral stenosis will greatly appreciate it if you can keep their heart rate low (Slow). You should also make it a goal to maintain the preload (Not too full), maintain the afterload (Not too tight), maintain the contractility (Not too strong), and keep them in normal sinus rhythm (Regular). MS: Make Slow.

Mitral Insufficiency – Hemodynamic Goals

Funny Nurse Forgot Reggie's Meds

Fast (increase heart rate)

Not too full (maintain to slightly increase preload)

Forward (decrease afterload)

Regular (maintain normal sinus rhythm)

Maintain contractility

It's important to consider many hemodynamic goals when it comes to patients with mitral insufficiency. While it's vital to keep their heart rate up (Fast), don't forget to maintain or even increase the preload (Not too full), decrease the afterload (Forward), maintain the contractility, and keep them in normal sinus rhythm (Regular). Try to avoid anything that would cause an increase in pulmonary vascular resistance. MI: Myocardial Increase.

Hypertrophic Cardiomyopathy – Hemodynamic Goals

My **F**ace **T**urns **R**ed **N**ightly

Maintain normal heart rate

Full (increased preload)

Tight (increased afterload)

Regular (normal sinus rhythm is crucial)

Not too strong (slightly depressed myocardial contractility)

Hypertrophic cardiomyopathy causes the heart to become thicker, thereby making it more difficult to pump blood through. For these patients, it's important to try to maintain a normal heart rate, keep the preload higher (Full), increase the afterload (Tight), and somewhat depressed contractility (Not too strong).

Idiopathic Hypertrophic Subaortic Stenosis (IHSS) - Changes that Increase Outflow Obstruction

II DD CHAP

Increased **C**ontractility

Increased **H**eart rate

Decreased **A**fterload

Decreased **P**reload

Idiopathic hypertrophic subaortic stenosis causes the left ventricle to become hypertrophied, narrowing the outflow tract and impeding left ventricle ejection. This can be made worse by increased contractility, increased heart rate, decreased afterload, and decreased preload. For these patients, try to maintain or slightly decrease contractility, decrease the heart rate, increase the afterload, and increase the preload.

Pulmonary Artery Catheter – Acceptable Insertion Sites

(In order of ease of insertion)

FEARS

Femoral veins.

External jugular

Antecubital—preferably basilic

Right internal jugular

Subclavian

When inserting a pulmonary artery catheter, several sites are acceptable for insertion. The femoral vein is the easiest place to put it, followed by the external jugular vein, the antecubital vein (basilic is preferred), the right internal jugular vein, and the subclavian vein. The left internal jugular vein should not be used as a site of insertion due to the increased incidence of possible complications.

Nervous System

Cerebral Perfusion Pressure (CPP) – Calculation

$$CPP = MAP - ICP$$

$$Candy = Mike - Ike$$

If you know the mean arterial pressure and the intracranial pressure, then you can easily figure out what the cerebral perfusion pressure is. Simply subtract the ICP from the MAP. This can also work in other ways. For example, you can figure out the MAP if you know what the CPP and the ICP is. You can also figure out what the ICP is if you know the CPP and the MAP. However, there is an exception to this rule. If the right atrial pressure (RAP) is abnormally elevated and higher than the intracranial pressure (ICP), then the cerebral perfusion pressure (CPP) = MAP-RAP, rather than MAP-ICP.

Electroconvulsive Therapy (ECT) – Drugs That Prolong Seizure Activity

CAKE

Caffeine, **C**lozapine

Aminophylline, **A**lfentanil

Ketamine

Etomidate

Electroconvulsive Therapy is commonly used to treat depression and other psychological issues, such as bipolar disorder. While we want these patients to be asleep and comfortable, we don't want to use medications that may depress seizure activity. In fact, some of the medications can actually prolong seizure activity. These include caffeine, clozapine, aminophylline, alfentanil, ketamine, and etomidate. These procedures are relatively short and typically do not require an endotracheal tube.

Increased Intracranial Pressure – Treatments During Anesthesia

CRASHED

Cerebral Vasoconstrictor/**C**ool the Patient

Restrict Fluids

Avoid Hypertension

Steroid

Hyperventilate

Elevate the Head

Dehydrate the Brain

The anesthetist has many options to treat increased intracranial pressure. A cerebral vasoconstrictor may be used, such as etomidate, thiopental, or Propofol. You might consider cooling the patient to 34 degrees Celsius, as this can help to protect the brain while surgery is going on. Fluids should be restricted as the patient's condition allows, and hypertension should be avoided. The brain can be dehydrated by using mannitol or Lasix. Hyperventilation should help by causing more cerebral vasoconstriction, while elevating the head of the bed to 30 degrees should help cerebral venous drainage. Steroids, such as dexamethasone, may be helpful in decreasing localized edema that is surrounding tumors.

Controlled Hypotension – Agents Used That Increase Intracranial Pressure (ICP)

NASH

Nitroglycerin

Adenosine
Sodium nitroprusside

Hydralazine

Sometimes, it's necessary to keep the patient's blood pressure lower in certain circumstances, often to prevent excessive bleeding. To accomplish this, controlled hypotension may be done. But the anesthesia provider should be aware of the ramifications of the medications given to accomplish this. Nitroglycerin, Adenosine, Sodium nitroprusside, and Hydralazine can all increase intracranial pressure while lowering the blood pressure. This is especially important to know because controlled hypotension is often done during neurological procedures.

Cervical Spine – Increased Risk for Potential Instability

NAILS

Neck pain

Any neurological signs or symptoms

Intoxication

Loss of consciousness at the scene

Severe distracting pain

When dealing with a trauma, ruling out a cervical spine injury is extremely important. But before you can get the patient to radiology to confirm anything, it would be a good idea to look at their symptoms. If they are having neck pain, you should investigate further. Are they intoxicated or are there any other neurological signs or symptoms? Is their pain severe and distracting? Was their loss of consciousness at the scene? All of these things make the patient at a greater risk for cervical spine instability.

Trigeminal Nerve – Branches

MOM

Maxillary

Ophthalmic

Mandibular

The trigeminal nerve, which just so happens to be cranial nerve V, provides sensory innervation to the region of the face. The three branches of the trigeminal nerve include the maxillary, ophthalmic, and mandibular. The mandibular branch provides both motor and sensory innervation, while the maxillary and ophthalmic branches provide only sensory innervation.

Brainstem Medulla – Centers

CVS CopyRight

Coughing

Vomiting

Swallowing

Cardiovascular

Respiratory

The brainstem consists of the pons, the midbrain, and the medulla oblongata. The medulla is the lower part of the brainstem connected to the spinal cord. It is responsible for coughing, vomiting, sneezing, and swallowing. It is also the portion of the brain that controls the cardiovascular and respiratory systems. Therefore, the medulla is what takes care of blood pressure, heart rate, and breathing.

Autonomic Hyperreflexia – Treatment

DVR

Deepening Anesthesia

Vasodilator

Removal of Stimulus

Autonomic hyperreflexia, also known as autonomic dysreflexia, typically happens with patients who have a spinal cord injury at T7 or above. Patients with other disorders, such as Guillain-Barré syndrome and multiple sclerosis, could also be susceptible. When these patients come in contact with certain stimuli, the nervous system may overreact, causing hypertension and tachycardia at first, with an extreme vagal response likely to follow shortly after. A common stimulus for this response is overdistension of the bladder.

If your patient has this type of response during surgery, the first step that has the highest chance of stopping it is to remove the stimulus causing it. If the bladder is distended, insert a catheter to drain it. If the surgeon is irrigating the bladder for a urology procedure, have them release some of the pressure. You can also try deepening the anesthesia, so the response isn't quite as profound. A vasodilator may be used if it continues (i.e. sodium nitroprusside).

Intracranial Pressure – IV Agents that Decrease ICP

<u>BEBOP</u>

Benzodiazepines

Etomidate

Barbiturates

Opioids

Propofol

Whether intended or not, several medications that we give have the ability to decrease intracranial pressure. These include benzodiazepines, such as versed, etomidate, and Propofol. It also happens with barbiturates, such as phenobarbital, and opioids, such as morphine.

Wake-up Test – Complications

DREAMS

Dislodgement of Instrumentation

Recall

Extubation

Air Embolus

Myocardial Ischemia

Self-injury

Wake-up tests are used in some neurosurgical cases to see if the patient is still neurologically intact during or after a critical point. When this is done, several complications are possible. For instance, any instrumentation the surgeon has in place may become dislodged. Although rare, the patient may have recall after the surgery is complete. If they move too much, they could possibly extubate themselves or cause accidental injury. If the patient takes a deep breath, they could get an air embolus from open venous sinuses.

Central Pontine Myelinolysis – Precipitating Situations

HOT

Head injury

Orthotopic liver transplantation

TURP syndrome

Central pontine myelinolysis is a neurological problem that usually happens after correction of hyponatremia. When it is corrected too rapidly with hypertonic saline, it can damage the myelin sheath of the brainstem (pons portion) nerve cells. These patients will have an altered level of consciousness, with eventual difficulty speaking and swallowing. If untreated, the patients can become paralyzed, "locked-in," and eventually die. Head injury, TURP syndrome, and orthotopic liver transplantation can all cause hyponatremia. Therefore, they are precipitating situations that could lead to CPM if the low sodium is treated too quickly.

Arnold-Chiari Malformation - Signs and Symptoms

ARDS

Apneic episodes

Recurrent aspiration

Difficulty swallowing

Stridor

Arnold-Chiari malformation is a condition that consists of the herniation of the cerebellar tonsils through the foramen magnum, often compressing the brainstem also. Common symptoms include episodes of apnea, recurrent aspiration, dysphagia, and stridor. These patients may also have frequent headaches, vomiting, neck pain, tinnitus, neuropathies, and scoliosis, among others.

Pediatrics/
Obstetrics

Persistent Fetal Circulation (Precipitating Factors)

Have **A** **H**elpful **P**ediatrician

Hypoxemia

Acidosis

Hypothermia

Pneumonia

You may recall that babies in utero have a different circulatory pattern. They are connected to the mother's blood by way of the umbilical cord. Blood comes through the umbilical cord and the ductus venosus shunts the oxygenated blood away from the liver and in the direction of the heart. This blood then goes through the inferior vena cava (IVC) into the right atrium. This blood then enters the left atrium via the foramen ovale, bypassing the lungs. The ductus arteriosus also shunts blood away from the lungs, into the aorta. This mixed blood then travels through the rest of the fetal body before going back to the placenta.

Once the baby is born, the umbilical cord gets clamped, interrupting this fetal blood flow. The baby starts to breathe and the lungs expand. The blood pressure increases and pulmonary pressures decrease, eventually leading to the closure of the foramen ovale and ductus arteriosus.

In persistent fetal circulation, there is increased pulmonary vascular resistance and right-to-left shunting, thereby preventing the normal circulatory changes from taking place. This can be common in preterm infants and infants with metabolic abnormalities such as sepsis, congenital diaphragmatic hernia, meconium aspiration, hypothermia, and asphyxia.

Fetal Circulation – 4 things that can compromise utero-placental blood flow

HEAL

Hypoxemia (maternal)

Excessive uterine activity

Aortocaval compression

Low blood pressure (maternal)

Fetal Circulation – 4 things that can improve utero-placental blood flow

FOME (Fear Of Missing Everything)

Fluids

Oxytocin infusion adjustment

Maternal position changes (to avoid aortocaval compression)

Ephedrine

Emergence Delirium in Children – Risk Factors

CAT CRAP

Child Temperament

Age

Type of Surgery

Characteristic of anesthetic

Rapid Emergence

Adjunct Medication

Preoperative Anxiety

Emergence delirium can happen with any child after receiving anesthesia. But certain characteristics may point to an increased likelihood of it happening. Children under five years old are more likely to experience emergence delirium, as are those with a poor temperament (poor socialization, difficulty adapting). It is more common after ophthalmologic and otolaryngologic surgeries and when adjunct medications, such as opioids, are used. You may also see it when the emergence from anesthesia is done rapidly or when the child is very anxious in pre-op. In most cases of emergence delirium, the child was anxious in the pre-operative area.

Inverted Uterus – Anesthetic Considerations

Baby **GROWL**

Blood Ready

General Anesthesia

Rapid Sequence Induction

Oxygen

Warm Fluids

Large Bore Catheters

An inverted uterus during vaginal delivery is a serious issue that must be taken care of quickly. For surgery, there are some anesthetic considerations that must be taken when you go back to the OR. The plan should include general anesthesia with a volatile anesthetic using rapid sequence induction. Once the ET tube is secured, place an OG tube to suction gastric contents. Have blood readily available and be prepared to give a lot of fluid through large bore IVs. Make sure the fluids are warmed to prevent hypothermia.

Uterine Atony - Anesthetic Management

V BOOT

Vital Signs

Blood Replacement

Oxygen

Oxytocin

Trendelenburg

Uterine tone and contraction are required to stop the bleeding after the birth of the baby. Uterine atony is when there is a loss of tone after delivery. This can be managed with medications, such as oxytocin, methergine, and hemabate. Blood loss should be replaced by crystalloids or colloids, followed by blood if necessary. You can try placing the patient in the Trendelenburg position and give oxygen by face mask. Monitor the vital sign closely, including central venous pressure to monitor fluid status if a central line is available.

Fetal Scalp Electrode Placement – Complications

SELLS

Sepsis

Ecchymoses

Lacerations

Leakage of cerebrospinal fluid

Scalp abscesses

A fetal scalp electrode is a wire that is used to closely and reliably monitor variability of fetal heart rate. Common complications of this practice include sepsis, ecchymosis, laceration, and leakage of CSF. However, the most common problem that happens is abscess on the scalp. There may also be complications for the mother, including damage to the vagina wall (i.e. laceration).

Coagulation/ Bleeding Disorders

Disseminated Intravascular Coagulation (DIC) - Treatment

People **C**ry **E**very **F**riday

Platelets

Cryoprecipitate

Eliminate the underlying cause

Fresh-frozen plasma

Disseminated Intravascular Coagulation (DIC) happens when excessive clotting is caused by some injury or disease. The clotting proteins may eventually get depleted, leading to excessive bleeding and organ injury. Treatment may include blood products, such as platelets, cryoprecipitate, and fresh-frozen plasma. Elimination of the underlying cause is paramount to recovery, but you may find yourself treating the symptoms as they come until that happens.

Blood Components - Four Most Commonly Administered

Poor People Cry Frequently

Packed red blood cells

Platelet concentrates

Cryoprecipitate

Fresh frozen plasma

As anesthesia providers, we administer many types of blood components. But the four most common are packed red blood cells, platelets, cryoprecipitate, and fresh frozen plasma. These are some of the types of questions you may see on boards.

Thromboelastography (TEG) – Parameters Measured

L MARK

LY30 (Clot Lysis)

MA (Maximum Amplitude)

Alpha angle (α)

R (Reaction Time)

K (Clot Formation Time)

Thromboelastography (TEG) is a good measurement to determine how well platelets are functioning, providing information on the quality, rather than just a number. It can be helpful in directing blood transfusion during certain surgeries, such as major trauma, cardiac, and liver transplantation. The five parameters that are monitored in a TEG include clot lysis, maximum amplitude, alpha angle, reaction time, and clot formation time.

The LY30 represents fibrinolysis as an equation, shown as a percent decrease in amplitude after maximum amplitude. MA represents maximum amplitude, the point at which the fibrin clot is the strongest. The alpha angle represents how quickly the clot forms. The reaction time (R) represents the amount of time it takes for the clot to begin to form. Finally, the clot formation time (K) represents the amount of time it takes for the clot to reach a specific strength, based on thrombin and platelet activation.

Pharmacology

Nondepolarizing Muscle Relaxants – Classification

Benzylisoquinoliniums

"**curium**"

Miva**curium**
Atra**curium**
Cisatra**curium**
Doxa**curium**
d-tubocurarine (exception – no longer used)
Metocurine (exception – no longer used)

Steroid Derivatives

"**curonium**"

Ve**curonium**
Ro**curonium**
Pan**curonium**
Pipe**curonium**

Clonidine – Clinical Uses

MOP HANDS

Myocardial ischemia protection
Opioid withdrawal
Preanesthetic medication

Hypertension
Adjunct to regional anesthesia
Neuraxial Analgesia
Diagnose pheochromocytoma
Shivering

Clonidine is an alpha-2 agonist, much like precedex, commonly used for sedation and hypertension. But it can also be useful for other things, such as myocardial ischemia protection in the intraoperative period, as a preanesthetic medication, an adjunct to regional anesthesia, and in spinals and epidurals. It can be helpful in patients who are withdrawing from opioids, taking much of the edge off and decreasing the withdrawal time for many of them. Clonidine is also helpful for shivering, which may be good postoperatively, by inhibiting thermoregulatory vasoconstriction. Finally, it can be an aid in diagnosing pheochromocytoma with the clonidine suppression test. When clonidine is given, catecholamine production is usually decreased. If this doesn't happen, then there is a high likelihood of pheochromocytoma.

Amide Toxicity – Potentiating Agents

Can't **P**rocess **A**mides

Cimetidine

Propranolol

Anesthetic gases

When we're talking about amide toxicity, we're talking about inhibition of our old friend, the cytochrome P450 system. Cimetidine, Propranolol, and volatile anesthetics are all examples of agents that potentiate amide toxicity. They inhibit the cytochrome P450 system, thereby decreasing the clearance of amides, causing buildup.

Local Anesthetics – Ways to Increase Potency

Help **C**rnas **E**levate **L**ocals

Halide to the aromatic ring

Carbon atoms

Ester linkage

Large alkyl group on the tertiary amide nitrogen

Lipid solubility and potency may be increased by adding things chemically. Try to stay awake while we go through a little chemistry. One way to increase potency is by adding a halide to the aromatic benzene ring. Examples of halides are chloride ions, bromide ions, etc. You can also add carbon atoms or an ester linkage. Lastly, you can add a large alkyl group to the tertiary amide nitrogen.

Anesthetic Dosing – Agents Dosed by Total Body Weight (in Obese Patients)

No **S**kinny **P**eople **D**oses

Neostigmine

Succinylcholine

Propofol

Dexmedetomidine

Some medications should be dosed by ideal body weight, based on the person's height. But some drugs that we give in anesthesia must be based on total body weight, taking every kilogram into account. Some of the medications include neostigmine, succinylcholine, Precedex, and Propofol (as a maintenance dose).

Statin Therapy – Adverse Effects

RICH GM

Rash

Increased liver enzymes

CNS dysfunction

Headache

Gastrointestinal distress

Muscle weakness

Although statin drugs are great for treating hyperlipidemia, they are not without problems. Some common adverse effects include rash, headache, gastrointestinal distress, increased liver enzymes, and hepatotoxicity. They may also cause neurological issues, such as severe depression, and muscle weakness or myalgia. A major concern is myopathy and the resulting rhabdomyolysis, which may eventually lead to death.

Glucagon Injection – Systemic Effects

RIP

Relaxes gastrointestinal smooth muscle

Increases myocardial contractility

Promotes glycogenolysis

Glucagon is often requested during certain surgeries due to various systemic effects. It relaxes gastrointestinal smooth muscle, which includes the sphincter of Oddi. This can help with the passing of bile stones. It also increases myocardial contractility, which can be useful after cardiac surgery or in cases of heart failure. Lastly, it promotes glycogenolysis, which may be used in cases of hypoglycemia.

Dose-response Curve - Descriptive Characteristics

PIES

Potency

Individual variability

Efficacy

Slope

If you're anything like me, your eyes begin to glaze over anytime you hear the words "dose-response curve." But it's something we should know since we give multiple drugs all day. This type of graph charts the dose of a particular drug on one axis and that drug's response on the other. Dose-response curves are differentiated by potency, individual variability, efficacy, and the slope of the curve. So this means there will be differences based on the strength of a drug, how each individual reacts, and how well it produced the desired effect.

Membrane Diffusion – Dependent Factors

Move That Lazy Crap

Molecular Weight
Thickness of Membrane
Lipid Solubility
Concentration Gradient

The diffusion of a drug across the cell membrane is dependent upon several factors. A substance with a high molecular weight will have a lower rate of diffusion than that a substance with a smaller molecular weight. The thicker the cell membrane, the lower the diffusion rate. The more lipid soluble a substance is, the higher the diffusion rate. Finally, the higher the concentration gradient, the greater the diffusion rate. Maybe this will help you remember:

MORE molecular weight = LOWER diffusion

MORE membrane thickness = LOWER diffusion

MORE lipid solubility = GREATER diffusion

MORE concentration gradient = GREATER diffusion

Intra-arterial Thiopental Injection – Signs and Symptoms

ABC

Arterial vasospasm

Blanching of skin

Cyanosis

Although thiopental is used less these days, it is still utilized in some places and still can show up on tests. If thiopental is accidentally injected into an artery, the patient will experience a few problems. They will likely have intense pain in the arm with arterial vasospasm. You may see distal pulses disappear and blanching of the skin. Finally, the patient could become cyanotic and the site of administration might eventually become gangrenous.

Naloxone – Opioid Actions Easily Reversed

PUN

Pruritus

Urinary retention

Nausea and vomiting

Naloxone – Opioid Actions Reversed with Higher Doses

Reverse Sandman

Respiratory Depression

Sedation (Profound)

Narcan is a great drug that can help reverse some of the effects from too much opioid. But some of these effects disappear more easily than others. Narcan doesn't have much of a problem taking away the itching, nausea, and urinary retention caused by opioids. However, it has a harder time reversing the profound sedative and respiratory depression effects. These symptoms may require higher doses to achieve the desired effect.

Plasma Cholinesterase – Conditions that Diminish its Activity

PLAY

Pregnancy

Liver disease

Atypical plasma cholinesterase

Young age

Succinylcholine and ester local anesthetics are metabolized by plasma cholinesterase. Therefore, diminishing plasma cholinesterase will prolong the action of these drugs. Keep this in mind when taking care of certain patients. It is diminished during pregnancy and in liver cirrhosis. It is also diminished in the first six months of life and if these patients have atypical plasma cholinesterase.

Non-Depolarizing Muscle Relaxants – Potentiating Drugs

CLAD

Calcium channel blockers

Local anesthetics

Aminoglycoside antibiotics

Dantrolene

Non-depolarizing muscle relaxants may be potentiated by certain medications, making them last longer than they normally would. This is true in the case of calcium channel blockers, local anesthetics, aminoglycoside antibiotics, and dantrolene. Keep this in mind when giving these paralytics to patients on these drugs and adjust the dosage accordingly.

Antimuscarinics – Administration Reasons

BIRDS

Bronchodilation

Increase Heart Rate

Reversal of Cholinergic Crisis

Decrease Airway Secretions

Sedation and Amnesia

Antimuscarinics are anticholinergics that block the muscarinic, rather than nicotinic, acetylcholine receptors. Some of the effects are desirable and some aren't, depending on the patient and the situation. Some of the reasons you might give antimuscarinics include bronchodilation, increase heart rate, reverse cholinergic crisis (atropine), sedation and amnesia (scopolamine), and to decrease airway secretions (antisialagogue effect).

Cholinesterase Inhibitors – Quaternary vs Tertiary

A **PEN** costs a **Quarter**

Pyridostigmine

Edrophonium

Neostigmine

are **Quater**nary ammonium substances, meaning they are charged and have four substituents.

PHYSics is **TER**rifying

Physostigmine

is a **Ter**tiary amine, meaning it is uncharged (so it readily crosses the blood-brain barrier) and has three substituents.

Class I Antiarrhythmics – Uses

SAW

Supraventricular dysrhythmias

Atrial fibrillation

Wolff-Parkinson-White syndrome

Antiarrhythmics are used to treat several abnormal cardiac rhythms and are divided into classes. Class I antiarrhythmics work primarily by blocking the sodium channel. They are often used to treat supraventricular and some ventricular dysrhythmias. They also have the ability to slow the atrial rate, which is helpful for atrial fibrillation. For patients with Wolff-Parkinson-White syndrome, these medications can help to suppress the tachyarrhythmias. Common drugs in this class include lidocaine, flecainide, phenytoin, and procainamide.

Calcium Channel Blockers – Uses

SAVE

Supraventricular tachydysrhythmias

Angina pectoris

Vasospasm

Essential Hypertension

Calcium channel blockers are separated into dihydropyridines and non-dihydropyridines, which are also subclassified into phenylalkylamines and benzothiazepines. They are commonly used to treat supraventricular tachyarrhythmias, hypertension, angina, coronary artery vasospasm, and cerebral artery vasospasm. Examples of dihydropyridines include drugs like amlodipine, nicardipine, and nifedipine. Verapamil is the only phenylalkylamine in use currently, while diltiazem is the only benzothiazepine in use currently.

Protamine – Adverse Effects

<u>SAP</u>

Systemic hypotension

Allergic reactions

Pulmonary hypertension

Protamine is used to reverse heparin by forming a stable complex that neutralizes its anticoagulant activity. The adverse effects from protamine administration are usually related to the histamine release it causes. You may see systemic hypotension, allergic reactions, or pulmonary hypertension. These may be exacerbated if pushed too quickly. Allergic reactions are more common in diabetic patients who take NPH insulin and men who have had a vasectomy.

Conversions

% to mg/mL

If you want to know the concentration of a drug, but all you have is the percent (%), it's simple to figure out how many milligrams (mg) there are per milliliter (mL). Simply move the decimal point to the right by one place. For example:

0.2%: 2 mg/mL

5%: 50 mg/mL

1:100,000 to mcg/mL

A simple shortcut for converting a 1:100,000 solution (or similar) to mcg/mL is to divide 1 million (1,000,000) by the denominator. For example:

1,000,000/100,000: 10 mcg/mL

Anaphylactic Reactions – Hypnotics Likely to Cause

Makes **T**hem **P**uffy

Midazolam

Thiopental

Propofol

Anaphylactic reactions are a cause for extreme concern, and many medications are known to provoke it. Three common hypnotics used in anesthesia are also more likely than others to cause anaphylaxis. Propofol is the most likely hypnotic medication to trigger such a reaction.

Anesthesia
Basics

Gas Cylinders – Amount Remaining

The amount remaining in the cylinder can be determined by the reading on the pressure gauge with these 4 gases:

NOAH

Nitrogen

Oxygen

Air

Helium

If gases are in liquid form in the cylinder, then the amount remaining cannot be ascertained simply by reading the pressure gauge. However, nitrogen, oxygen, air, and helium are all gases that are not in liquid form in high pressure cylinders. Therefore, you can determine the amount remaining by reading the pressure gauge.

Orbital Muscles

IS SLIM

Inferior Rectus

Superior Rectus

Superior Oblique

Lateral Rectus

Inferior Oblique

Medial Rectus

Inferior Rectus: look down (Cranial nerve III – oculomotor)
Superior Rectus: look up (Cranial nerve III – oculomotor)

Superior Oblique: look in and down (Cranial nerve IV – trochlear)
Lateral Rectus: look outward (Cranial nerve VI – abducens)
Inferior Oblique: look out and up (Cranial nerve III – oculomotor)
Medial Rectus: look inward (Cranial nerve III – oculomotor)

Aldrete's Scoring System – Criteria

ARCCC

Activity

Respiration

Circulation

Consciousness

Color

The Aldrete's scoring system is used by the post-anesthesia care unit to determine when it's safe to discharge the patient to the next phase. The five criteria that comprise this system include activity, respiration, circulation, consciousness, and color. Each of these is worth 0 to 2 points and patients can be discharged when their score is greater than 8. However, they may be kept longer if the nurses and doctors deem it necessary.

Medical Negligence Action - Elements

Dumb **B**oys **D**on't **C**all

Duty

Breach of Duty

Damage

Cause

If a plaintiff brings forth a medical negligence action, they must prove that duty, breach of duty, damage, and 'cause' all existed in their case. Duty means that a reasonable standard of care was expected. Breach of duty means that this standard was not met in some way. Damage means that physical or emotional injury occurred. Cause means that the damage was caused by the defendant. The damage to the plaintiff must be a direct result of the defendant's action.

MRI Contraindications – Implanted Devices

CAB

Cardiac pacemakers

AICD

Biological pumps

Any object with a high susceptibility to magnetization could place the patient or that object at risk during an MRI. Biological pumps, such as implanted pain pumps and insulin pumps, may get damaged or cause harm to the patient. The same can be said for pacemakers and AICDs, which may convert to asynchronous mode, be deactivated, or get switch damage. MRIs may also be contraindicated in patients with vascular clips, stents, and wire-spiraled endotracheal tubes.

Soda Lime Exhaustion - Indicators

FAITH

Flushed dry skin

Absorbent turns color

Inspired CO2 concentration increases

Tachycardia

Hypertension

When the patient is showing any signs of increased CO2 production, then you might want to take a look at your soda lime canister to see if it needs to be changed. Common signs of soda lime exhaustion include flushed dry skin, tachycardia, and hypertension. The easiest way to tell though, is by looking at your CO2 waveform and the canister itself. If the patient is rebreathing CO2, the absorbent has changed color, and there is a large amount of condensation in the canister, then the soda lime has probably been exhausted. Get a new one!

Awareness During Anesthesia – Increased Risk

PITA (Pain In The Ass)

Provider abuse of anesthetic drugs

Inhalational agent not turned on/empty vaporizer

TIVA not begun or failure of device

Anesthesia discontinued too early

Awareness during anesthesia can be a very scary thing for our patients. One of the most asked questions in the pre-operative area is "how do you know if I'm asleep enough?" Although a rare occurrence, there are some things that may increase the risk of awareness. If the anesthesia provider is abusing the anesthetics, then they may charge some drugs to the patient but never administer them, instead pocketing them for later. The anesthetist may forget to turn on the gas or simply forget to fill the vaporizer. Another problem may occur during a TIVA when gas can't be used. After induction, the IV meds may be forgotten (since the anesthetist is used to turning on the gas, rather than starting a pump). Lastly, anesthesia may be discontinued too early. As the surgery is ending, the anesthetist may cut the gas too early in trying to achieve "the perfect wakeup."

Volatile Anesthetics – Renal Changes

RUG

Renal blood flow

Urine output

Glomerular filtration rate

Volatile anesthetics can affect many body systems in various ways, and the kidneys are no exception. They can cause decreases in renal blood flow, urine output, and glomerular filtration rate. Desflurane may be a better choice in patients with already impaired renal function.

Gamma Amino Butyric Acid Type A (GABA_A) Receptor – Ligand Binding Sites

GABAS **P**ossessive **B**inding **P**laces

G

Anesthetics

Barbiturates

Alcohol

Steroids

Propofol

Benzodiazepines

Picrotoxin

We should all be familiar with the name gamma amino butyric acid (GABA), since it is believed to have much to do with the function of anesthesia. If you look closely, you'll see that five of these sites involve anesthesia. GABA Type A ligand binding sites include anesthetics, barbiturates, alcohol, steroids, Propofol, benzodiazepines, and picrotoxin.

Heat Loss – Causes (Most to Least)

Really Cover Every Corner

Radiation >

Convection >

Evaporation >

Conduction

As anesthesia providers, we're responsible for the maintenance of patient temperature, making sure they don't get hypothermic. Therefore, it's important to know how heat is lost so we can figure out ways to stop it. During anesthesia, heat is mostly lost through radiation, which is the transfer of heat from the body to other cooler things nearby. The patient loses heat when the ambient temperature in the operating room is too low. Convection happens when forced air flows over exposed skin and removes heat along with it. Heat is lost by evaporation through use of surgical prep solutions and open cavities in the body. Conduction is when heat gets transferred from the body to a surface it is in contact with, such as the cold operating room bed.

Volatile Inhaled Agents – Trade Names

HF – **H**epatic **F**ailure

EE – **E**vil **E**mpire

IF – **I** **F**arted

DS – **D**ark **S**ide

SU – **S**uck **U**p

Halothane is **F**luothane™

Enflurane is **E**thrane™

Isoflurane is **F**orane™

Desflurane is **S**uprane™

Sevoflurane is **U**ltane™

Nitrous Oxide (N₂O) – Side Effects

<u>CACA</u>

Congenital anomalies

Aplastic anemia

CNS toxicity

Abortion (Spontaneous)

As we all know, nitrous oxide isn't without serious side effects. For instance, it is known to cause nausea and can also get trapped in closed air spaces, so should be avoided in certain patients. It may cause spontaneous abortion or congenital anomalies, so avoid or use caution in pregnant patients, particularly during organogenesis. Nitrous oxides could also cause central nervous system toxicity and aplastic anemia. Although it can be a very useful drug, be cautious when administering and make sure you think before you turn that dial.

Anesthetic Brain Uptake – Dependent Factors

Anesthesia **I**s **B**riskly **C**hanging

Alveolar Ventilation

Inspired Concentration

Blood Solubility

Cardiac Output

The uptake of volatile anesthetics by the brain is dependent upon several factors. The higher the alveolar ventilation, the faster the uptake. The more you increase the inspired concentration, the faster the uptake. The more blood soluble a gas is, the slower the uptake, due to the slower rise in alveolar partial pressure. Finally, when a patient has a lower cardiac output, it increases the uptake to the brain.

HIGHER Alveolar ventilation = FASTER uptake

HIGHER Inspired concentration = FASTER uptake

HIGHER Blood solubility = SLOWER uptake

HIGHER Cardiac output = SLOWER uptake

Complications
/ Disorders

Fluid Overload in the TURP Patient – Late Signs

DASH

Dyspnea

Arrhythmias

Seizures

Hyponatremia (severe)/ **H**ypotension

When a patient is undergoing a TURP procedure, fluid overload is a potential complication due to the large amount of fluid used during surgery. These can lead to several problems, but later signs include shortness of breath, arrhythmias, seizures, hypotension, and severe hyponatremia. Most of the problems arise because of the dilution of the sodium in the body.

Delayed Gastric Emptying – Possible Causes

<u>POOP</u> a <u>TAD</u>

Pregnancy
Obesity
Opioids
Pain

Trauma
Anxiety
Diabetes

When your patient has delayed gastric emptying, it puts them at a much higher risk for aspiration and PONV. Therefore, it's important to identify them pre-operatively. Some common causes include obesity, opioid use, pain, anxiety, and trauma. Patients who have been involved in a trauma should be considered NPO only up until the time of the trauma. If they had lunch at 1200, and they get in a car accident at 1500, they should be considered NPO for 3 hours, even if surgery isn't until 2000. The obvious causes for delayed gastric emptying are diabetes and pregnancy. Take caution with these patients.

Carcinoid Syndrome – Overproduced Hormonal Mediators

Some Penises Have Bumpy Knots

Serotonin

Prostaglandins

Histamine

Bradykinin

Kallikrein

Carcinoid syndrome happens because of carcinoid tumors, which most often present in the lungs or the digestive tract. It can cause overproduction of several hormonal mediators, including prostaglandins, histamine, bradykinin, and kallikrein. But the hallmark of carcinoid syndrome is serotonin overproduction. These produce several signs and symptoms, such as flushing and diarrhea. If the tumors are present in the lungs, you may also see dyspnea, chest pain, wheezing, or weight gain. If the tumors are present in the digestive tract, you could see abdominal pain, rectal pain and bleeding, bowel obstruction, or nausea.

Myotonic Dystrophy – Anesthetic Concerns

CRAP

Cardiomyopathy

Respiratory muscle weakness

Aspiration of gastric contents

Potential for abnormal responses to anesthetic drugs

Myotonic dystrophy is an inherited disorder and causes progressive muscle weakness. This creates cause for concern for the anesthetist in a variety of ways. These patients may present with arrhythmias, cardiomyopathy, and congestive heart failure. They may also have respiratory muscle weakness, so be cautious when using drugs that may cause respiratory depression. Myotonic dystrophy may cause decreased GI motility and lower esophageal sphincter tone, putting them at risk for aspiration. You may want to consider rapid sequence. You should also keep in mind that the reactions to anesthetic medications may not be as expected.

TURP – Glycine Side Effects

ANTHEM

Ammonia toxicity

Nausea and vomiting

Transient blindness

Headache

ECG changes

Myocardial depression

Transurethral resection of the prostate (TURP) involves the use of an irrigating agent, each with its own set of complications. If the surgeon uses glycine, it may lead to ammonia toxicity, nausea and vomiting, headache, ectopy, myocardial depression, and blindness (that typically resolves). The patient may also experience loss of light and accommodation reflexes. This is all in addition to the already present risk of fluid overload. Having the patient awake, using regional anesthesia, may help identify some of these symptoms earlier, allowing for quicker treatment.

Malignant Hyperthermia – Complications After it's Controlled

Rx MEDS

Recurrence

Myoglobinuric renal failure

Electrolyte abnormalities

Disseminated intravascular coagulation (DIC)

Skeletal muscle weakness

Malignant hyperthermia is a very dangerous potential complication of general anesthesia. If the patient is lucky enough to survive the initial attack, there are still several hurdles they will encounter before they are out of the woods. Recurrence of MH is a very strong possibility. The patient may also have myoglobinuric renal failure due to rhabdomyolysis, electrolyte abnormalities, skeletal muscle weakness, and DIC. All of this is caused by the calcium buildup in the skeletal muscle. Assuming Dantrolene was given, this should be continued as recommended in the post-operative period.

Malignant Hyperthermia – Active Cooling Methods

Ice Cold Life Support

Intravenous normal saline

Cardiopulmonary bypass (in severe cases)

Lavage

Surface cooling

Malignant hyperthermia is a rare problem that anesthetists pray they will never have to come across. However, if it does happen, there are ways you can help actively cool the patient while giving the dantrolene. Chilled normal saline can be given intravenously. Lavage is also an option, using the orogastric route, urinary bladder, or into any open cavities. Ice packs should be placed at the patient's groin, neck, and axilla. Forced-air blankets that blow cold can also be implemented. In severe cases, cardiopulmonary bypass may be necessary to allow for cooling.

Mandibular Hypoplasia – Associated Congenital Diseases

PG Television

Pierre Robin Syndrome

Goldenhar Syndrome

Treacher Collins Syndrome

Mandibular hypoplasia is a condition that often causes an abnormal airway, making it more difficult to intubate. Three examples of congenital mandibular hypoplasia include Pierre Robin Syndrome, Goldenhar Syndrome, and Treacher Collins Syndrome. Although they are considered a difficult airway, these patients are often intubated after they go to sleep. Awake fiber optic intubation can be used, but it may do more harm than good. It can cause severe damage to the upper airway and they are still at risk for aspiration.

Chronic Alcoholics - Hematologic Abnormalities

Apparent Liver Trouble

Anemia

Leukopenia

Thrombocytopenia

Chronic alcoholics slowly, but surely, cause damage their liver that will usually kill them eventually if they don't stop drinking. This liver damage can lead to several hematologic abnormalities, including anemia, leukopenia, and thrombocytopenia. These patients are at a higher risk for bleeding, so keep that in mind during high risk surgeries. Medications that can worsen the liver damage should be avoided unless the benefits outweigh the risks.

Bladder Perforation – Signs and Symptoms

BAD HANDS

Bradycardia

Anxiety

Diaphoresis

Hypotension/Hiccups

Abdominal pain

Nausea

Dyspnea

Shoulder pain

Bladder perforation typically happens for 2 reasons: either it gets way overdistended or something punctures it. For example, in a TURP procedure, the irrigation fluid may cause too much pressure until the bladder wall can no longer hold. It may also happen if the surgeon accidentally hits the bladder with the resectoscope.

Bladder perforation may be intraperitoneal, extraperitoneal, or both. Intraperitoneal perforation usually happens in the dome of the bladder and may cause pain in the precordial area, shoulder, upper abdomen, or neck. Extraperitoneal perforation usually happens in the base of the bladder and may cause lower abdominal distention and pain in the inguinal, periumbilical, or suprapubic areas. Patients with bladder perforation may also have bradycardia, anxiety, diaphoresis, hypotension, hiccups, nausea, and shortness of breath.

Lower Esophageal Sphincter Tone – Factors That Decrease

G SHOP

Glucagon

Secretin

Hiatal hernia

Obesity

Pregnancy

Lower esophageal sphincter tone is important because it helps prevent stomach contents from going up back into the esophagus. When the LES tone is lower, stomach contents are much more likely to re-enter the esophagus. This is important for us to know in anesthesia because a decreased LES tone greatly increases the risk for aspiration. You may want to consider doing a rapid sequence induction in these patients. Lower esophageal sphincter tone is decreased by many things, including pregnancy, obesity, hiatal hernia, secretin, and glucagon.

Glucose-6-phosphate-dehydrogenase (G6PDH) Deficiency – Drugs to Avoid

<u>MD NAPS</u>

Methylene blue

Doxorubicin

Nitroprusside

Aspirin

Penicillin/**P**rilocaine

Streptomycin/**S**ulfonamides

Glucose-6-phosphate-dehydrogenase (G6PDH) deficiency causes the breakdown of red blood cells. Although patients with this disorder often don't have any symptoms, it is not uncommon for them to experience malaise, dyspnea, dark urine, and jaundice. Medications that may trigger an episode should be avoided if possible. Some of these include methylene blue, doxorubicin, nitroprusside, aspirin, penicillin, prilocaine, streptomycin, and sulfonamides.

Duchenne Muscular Dystrophy – Anesthetic Concerns

CURDS

Cardiac arrest upon induction

Unpredictable susceptibility to malignant hyperthermia

Retention of pulmonary secretions

Delayed gastric emptying

Succinylcholine-induced hyperkalemia

Duchenne muscular dystrophy is a progressive disorder that causes the muscles to become weaker as time goes by. It is first diagnosed in childhood and affects primarily males. Because of the nature of the disease, we must be vigilant as anesthesia providers in anticipating certain complications. These patients have weakened heart muscle, so it is possible for them to go into cardiac arrest during the stress of induction. Also, because it is a muscular disorder, they may be more susceptible to malignant hyperthermia. They might have delayed gastric emptying and retention of pulmonary secretions, and they may be more difficult to extubate due to weakened breathing muscles. Be aware of the possibility of increased potassium after succinylcholine administration, even more so than the usual response.

Syndrome of Inappropriate ADH Secretion (SIADH) – Causes

CHIP

Carcinoma of the lung

Hypothyroidism

Intracranial tumors

Porphyria

In Syndrome of Inappropriate ADH Secretion (SIADH), too much ADH is being released into the body, causing too much fluid to be retained. This leads to dilution of sodium and resultant hyponatremia. Common causes include lung cancer or disease, hypothyroidism, brain tumors, and porphyria. The most common reason for SIADH is intracranial tumors. The hyponatremia and fluid overload in these patients may cause nausea, muscle weakness, tremors, shortness of breath, confusion, seizures, coma, and even death if left untreated.

Syndrome of Inappropriate ADH Secretion - Treatment

CHAR

Correct underlying cause

Hyperosmotic saline

Antagonize the effects of ADH

Restrict water intake

In Syndrome of Inappropriate ADH Secretion (SIADH), too much ADH is being released into the body, causing too much fluid to be retained. This leads to dilution of sodium and resultant hyponatremia. Common causes include lung cancer or disease, hypothyroidism, brain tumors, and porphyria. The hyponatremia and fluid overload in these patients may cause nausea, muscle weakness, tremors, shortness of breath, confusion, seizures, coma, and even death. Treatment should be first directed at correcting the underlying problem. Otherwise, you'll end up just chasing the symptoms. You can also give hyperosmotic saline (can be given with or without diuretics), restrict the intake of water, and give demecolcine. Demecolcine can antagonize the ADH effects on the renal tubule.

Diabetic Autonomic Neuropathy – Anesthetic Concerns

POG

Painless myocardial infarction

Orthostatic hypotension

Gastroparesis

Diabetic autonomic neuropathy affects the nervous system throughout the body, typically caused by poor glucose control. The nerves become damaged and are unable to function properly. These patients often have difficulty sensing feeling in their feet and may have poor eyesight. Gastroparesis is common, and the delayed gastric emptying puts them at a greater risk for aspiration. They may also be more likely to have silent heart attacks and orthostatic hypotension. Be ready with vasopressors, as they tend to need more support than patients without autonomic neuropathy.

Pheochromocytoma – Signs and Symptoms

Hormone-Discharging Tumor

Hypertension/**H**eadache

Diaphoresis

Tachycardia

A pheochromocytoma is a tumor located on the adrenal gland, specifically arising from the chromaffin cells. It stores and is capable of secreting catecholamines, sometimes in very large amounts. This causes hypertension, tachycardia, and diaphoresis. These patients often complain of a headache. The tumor is usually only located on one adrenal gland or the other, but it is seen bilaterally in some cases. Nonselective beta blockers should be avoided without proper alpha blockade also. Doing so could leave the vasoconstriction of alpha receptors unopposed without the beta-2 vasodilation.

Chronic Renal Failure - Pathophysiological Consequences

(in addition to electrolyte disturbances)

CHAMPS

Coagulopathies

Hypertension

Anemia

Metabolic acidosis

Pruritus

Susceptibility to infection

We all know about the electrolyte disturbances that may be present in patients with chronic renal failure. But we should also keep in mind the other problems that may arise from this condition. These patients are usually fluid overloaded and unable to clear a lot of the toxins that are normally excreted in the urine. Coagulopathies, high blood pressure, anemia, and pruritus are not uncommon. They are also more susceptible to infections. Don't forget about the metabolic acidosis that may be caused by the fluid and electrolyte shifts.

Complex Regional Pain Syndrome (CRPS) – Signs and Symptoms

ASSHAT

Active and Passive Motor Disorders

Sympathetic Dysfunction

Spontaneous Pain

Hyperalgia

Allodynia

Trophic, Sudomotor, Vasomotor Abnormalities

Complex Regional Pain Syndrome (CRPS) is a group of conditions that cause pain and swelling, usually starting in an arm or leg. It may start after some sort of trauma or injury and may affect the entire body in some patients. Some of the signs and symptoms to remember include active and passive motor disorders, hyperalgesia, and allodynia. These patients can also have sympathetic dysfunction, which may be seen as swelling and cyanosis. Pain can present spontaneously, without anything bringing it on. They may also have trophic, vasomotor and sudomotor (sweat gland) abnormalities. It is considered Type I CRPS if there is no evidence of nerve damage to the limb, while it is considered Type II if there is evidence of nerve damage in the limb.

Prune-belly Syndrome – Congenital Anomalies

Unstable Abdominal Condition

Urinary tract abnormalities

Absent abdominal wall muscles

Cryptorchidism

Prune-belly syndrome is a rare inherited disorder that causes problems with the urinary system. This condition can sometimes create areas of wrinkled skin on the stomach, which is where it gets its name. There are no associated problems with the gastrointestinal system. Instead, it is known for a triad of anomalies, including undescended testes (cryptorchidism), absent or partially absent abdominal wall muscles, and urinary tract abnormalities. These patients can also have club foot, ventricular septal defect, frequent UTIs, and musculoskeletal abnormalities.

Burns – Fluid Resuscitation (PA Cath Parameters)

Cool Mo Fos

Cardiac output

Mixed venous oxygen tension

Filling pressures

After a burn injury, administration of fluids is paramount in the initial phase. Fluids should be titrated according to specific goals, as outlined in formulas such as the Parke or modified Brooke. These goals can be monitored easily by using a pulmonary artery catheter. Fluid resuscitation can be shown to be adequate by reaching an acceptable cardiac output, mixed venous oxygen tension, and filling pressures.

Monitoring and Equipment

Medical Gas Lines - Common Contaminants

B WORM

Bacteria

Water

Oil

Residual sterilizing solutions.

Matter

Although medical gas lines are inspected for safety and contaminants, many things are often missed, due to inexperience and lack of expertise. Water is the most common contaminant, but there has also been reports of oil, bacteria, and particulate matter, such as dirt, sand, gravel, and dust. Sterilizing solutions have also been found, left as residual from previous use. These contaminants often enter during the initial construction of the pipelines. Anesthesia providers should make themselves aware of the safety code and be able to give input during construction. If already contaminated, the pipelines should be cleaned or purged.

Modern Vaporizers – Hazards

LOITER

Leaks

Overfilling with agent

Incorrect agent administration

Tipping

Reliance on breath-by-breath gas analysis

Over the years, anesthesia vaporizers have undergone many changes and technological advancements to improve the way we deliver care. But even today, there are still some hazards that they can present. Vaporizers can still leak and have electronic failures. There is nothing to prevent you from overfilling them with agents. It may be possible to fill certain ones with the wrong agent still, and there is also a heavy reliance now on breath-by-breath gas analysis, rather than preventative maintenance to keep problems from happening.

Proportion-Limiting Systems – Conditions That Can "Fool" Them

WILD

Wrong supply gas

Inert gas administration

Leaks downstream

Defective pneumatics or mechanics

Dilution of inspired oxygen concentration

In anesthesia workstations equipped with proportioning systems, hypoxic gas mixtures may be delivered in certain conditions. This includes the wrong supply gas, inert gas administration, downstream leaks, defective mechanics/pneumatics, or dilution of inspired oxygen concentration by volatile anesthetics.

Required Monitors on the Anesthesia Workstation

BIO HEAP

Blood pressure

Inspired Oxygen

Oxygen Supply Failure Alarm

Hypoxic guard system

Electrocardiogram (ECG)

Anesthetic Vapor Concentration

Pulse Oximetry

BIO HEAP is a good way to remember the basic required monitors on an anesthesia workstation. Blood pressure monitoring is a must, as is an inspired oxygen alarm, which must alarm within 30 seconds after the oxygen being delivered goes under 18%. There has to be an oxygen supply failure alarm and a hypoxic guard system that stops you from going under 21% oxygen when using nitrous. Lastly, the anesthesia workstation must have ecg monitoring, pulse oximetry, and anesthesia vapor concentration.

Regional
Anesthesia

Stellate Ganglion Blockade (Horner's Syndrome) - Signs and Symptoms

FACES

Flushing

Anhidrosis

Congestion

Eyes

Skin temperature increased

A stellate ganglion block is done to blunt the sympathetic system on the ipsilateral side of the arm and the face. Horner's syndrome indicates that a successful blockade has occurred. Signs and symptoms of Horner's Syndrome include facial and arm flushing (vasodilation), anhidrosis (lack of sweating), nasal congestion, ptosis, miosis, and increased skin temperature.

Neuraxial Block – Dyspnea Causes

PHAT

Position

Hypotension

Abdominal and intercostal muscles blockade

Thoracic proprioception blunting

During a spinal or epidural, dyspnea is a fairly common complication. There may be several possible causes for this, but the most common is hypotension. This is because the decreased blood pressure causes hypoperfusion in the brainstem. So if someone complains of shortness of breath after a neuraxial block, the first thought should be low blood pressure. However, it can also be caused by other things, such as simple positioning, when the abdominal contents are pressing up against the diaphragm. Dyspnea may also be due to a partial block of the abdominal and intercostal muscles. Finally, there may also be blunting of thoracic proprioception, in which patients have difficulty "feeling" the chest wall moving while taking a breath.

Spinal and Epidural Opioids – Side Effects

LINEUPS

Late respiratory depression

Ileus

Nausea and vomiting

Early respiratory depression

Urinary retention

Pruritus

Sedation

Giving opioids via epidural or spinal is not without potential side effects and complications. The thing you might worry about the most is delayed respiratory depression. But, don't forget about nausea, vomiting, itching, sedation, urinary retention, and eventual ileus down the road. Early respiratory depression is one of the least likely complications to arise.

High Spinal Anesthesia – Signs and Symptoms

HAND

Hypotension

Apnea

Nausea and vomiting

Dyspnea

A high spinal happens when the amount of medication is overestimated for the patient, resulting in a block above the desired level (usually T4). The reaction can vary in severity depending on how high it goes. Some common signs and symptoms include hypotension, shortness of breath, nausea, vomiting, and even respiratory failure. If it goes high enough, it could become a total spinal, causing the patient to lose consciousness. Cardiac arrest and death could follow if not dealt with quickly.

Retrobulbar Block – Desired Effects

AAA

Akinesia of the eye

Anesthesia of the eye

Abolishment of the oculo-cardiac reflex

The retrobulbar space is the area that is behind the globe of the eye. A retrobulbar block is done for eye surgeries, most often for cataract correction. A desired block will produce akinesia of the extraocular muscles, abolishment of the oculo-cardiac reflex, and anesthesia of the conjunctiva, cornea, and uvea.

Surgical
Procedures

Mediastinoscopy - Relative Contraindications

CATS

Cerebrovascular disease

Aortic aneurysm (thoracic)

Tracheal deviation

Superior vena cava obstruction

Mediastinoscopy is typically done to get lymph node biopsies to help stage lung cancer. It may also be done to aid in the diagnosis of other conditions like lymphoma or sarcoidosis. Relative contraindications include cerebrovascular disease, thoracic aortic aneurysm, tracheal deviation, and SVC obstruction. If the benefits outweigh the risks, then proceed with great caution in these cases. You don't want to end up with a complication like a stroke or aneurysm rupture.

LeFort III Fracture – Important Considerations

TIP

Tracheostomy

Intubation

Positioning

A Lefort III fracture is when all of the facial bones separate away from the cranial base, along with fractures of zygoma, nasal, and maxilla bones. These patients often have very limited mouth opening and instability of the facial structures, making intubation a challenge. After positioning optimally, consider an awake fiberoptic intubation. Another option is to go straight to a tracheostomy under local only anesthesia. Cricothyrotomy should be anticipated, but only done in case of emergency.

Mediastinoscopy – Vessels That Can Be Compressed

SIC

Subclavian Arteries

Innominate Artery

Carotid Arteries

Mediastinoscopy is typically done to get lymph node biopsies to help stage lung cancer. It may also be done to aid in the diagnosis of other conditions like lymphoma or sarcoidosis. During this procedure, the subclavian arteries, carotid arteries, and the innominate artery may be compressed. If the innominate artery is compressed, it will cause reduced blood flow through the right carotid and right subclavian arteries. It can also cause a decrease in cerebral perfusion, as can direct compression of the carotid arteries, especially in patients with cerebral vascular disease. If the right subclavian artery is directly or indirectly compressed, it will decrease the pressure and pulse in the right arm. It might be a good idea to place the pulse on on the right hand to monitor for this.

Strabismus Repair – Anesthetic Concerns

COMP

Cardiovascular effects of ocular medications

Oculo-cardiac reflex

Malignant hyperthermia

Postoperative nausea and vomiting

Strabismus repair involves working on the extraocular muscles to correct the underlying problem. But a seemingly simple surgery like this isn't quite so simple when you consider the possible complications. Since the surgeon will be working within the eye, the oculo-cardiac reflex is very much in play (remember the 'five and dime' mnemonic, involving the 5th and 10th cranial nerves). So watch out for bradycardia and nausea and vomiting. You should also be aware of the cardiovascular effects many of the ocular medications have, including CHF and arrhythmias. Patients with strabismus are more likely to have an underlying myopathy, therefore putting them at a greater chance of malignant hyperthermia happening. Stay away from succinylcholine in these patients (to avoid MH and increased intraocular pressure) and consider TIVA (which will also help with the PONV).

Radical Neck Dissection - Intraoperative Complications

BAM

Baroreceptors

Air embolism

Mainstem

Radical neck dissections are done to treat cancers or to prevent the spread of certain cancers. There are a number of possible complications, including but not limited to, baroreceptor compression, air embolism, and inadvertent mainstem intubation. When the baroreceptors are stimulated, the baroreceptor reflex is often initiated, causing bradycardia and hypotension. Because of positioning and manipulation of the head and neck, the endotracheal tube may migrate downward into the mainstem bronchus. This can be monitored for by checking bilateral breath sounds, peak inspiratory pressures, and the CO_2 waveform.

Patho-
physiology

Oxyhemoglobin Dissociation Curve - Rightward Shift Causes

2 TAPS

Increased **2**,3-DPG

Increased **T**emperature

Increased (**A**cidity) H+ concentration (decreased pH)

Increased **P**artial pressure of CO_2

Sickle cell disease

When the oxyhemoglobin dissociation curve shifts leftward, the hemoglobin tends to hold on to the oxygen more tightly. When it shifts rightward, the hemoglobin tends to release more oxygen to the tissues. A rightward shift is caused by increased temperature, acidity, partial pressure of carbon dioxide, and 2,3 DPG. It is also caused by sickle cell disease. Try to remember that when metabolism is increased, the curve shifts more to the right. In opposite conditions, it shifts to the left.

Adrenal Medulla – Catecholamines Secreted

END

Epinephrine

Norepinephrine

Dopamine

The adrenal medulla is controlled by the sympathetic nervous system and the hormones secreted by it create the "flight or fight" response. The two main catecholamines secreted are epinephrine and norepinephrine, but also dopamine in smaller amounts.

Natriuretic Peptides

CUBA

CNP (C-Type)

Urodilatin

BNP (Brain/B-Type)

ANP (Atrial/A-Type)

Peptides that cause the kidneys to excrete sodium (natriuresis) are called natriuretic peptides. ANP gets released from atrial muscle when the local walls stretch and when there is increased atrial volume. BNP gets released when ventricular muscle is distended. CNP gets released from the endothelium of major vessels in response to stress and other stimuli. Urodilatin is produced in the lower urinary tract and is excreted when mean arterial pressure (MAP) is increased or blood volume is increased. Natriuretic receptor-A binds ANP and BNP, while natriuretic receptor-B binds CNP.

Immunoglobulins

GAMED

Ig**G**

Ig**A**

Ig**M**

Ig**E**

Ig**D**

Immunoglobulins are basically antibodies that are able to recognize certain antigens, bind to them, and help to destroy them. IgG is found in all fluids in the body and is the most common type, making up around 75% of all serum antibodies. IgA is found mostly in mucous membranes, such as saliva, tears, and respiratory and gastrointestinal tracts. IgM is in the blood and lymph and is the first attacker of an infection. IgE is located in the skin, mucous membranes, and lungs. It is produced when there is an allergen, creating an allergic reaction. Finally, IgD is located in the blood in small amounts and is also co-expressed with IgM.

Signal Transduction Systems - Components

PEERS

Protein

Enzyme

External Signal

Receptor

Second Messenger

Signal transduction is the transfer of signals from the outside of a cell to the inside through its membrane. In this type of system, the first messengers (ligands) are external signals. Primary effectors are activated by the receptors, which are called signal transducers. An enzyme gets coupled to the receptor by a protein. The second messenger is an intracellular chemical that is promoted by an enzyme. The secondary effectors are activated by the second messengers.